WK
LOO
3/06.

Clinical
Endocrinology and

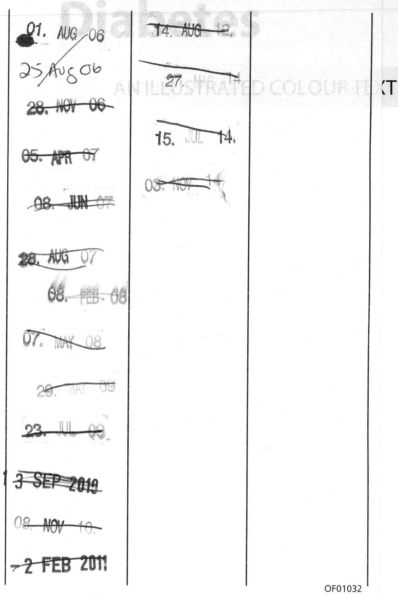

Diabetes

AN ILLUSTRATED COLOUR TEXT

01. AUG 06

25/Aug 06

28. NOV 06

05. APR 07

08. JUN 07

28. AUG 07

08. FEB 08

07. MAY 08

29. MAY 09

23. JUL 09

13 SEP 2010

08. NOV 10.

-2 FEB 2011

14. AUG 12.

27

15. JUL 14.

03. NOV 14

Commissioning Editor: Michael Parkinson
Project Development Manager: Clive Hewat
Project Manager: Nancy Arnott
Designer: Erik Bigland

Clinical Endocrinology and Diabetes

AN ILLUSTRATED COLOUR TEXT

Shern L. Chew BSc MD FRCP
Professor of Endocrine Medicine/Consultant Physician
Department of Endocrinology, St Bartholomew's and Royal
London School of Medicine, London, UK

David Leslie MD FRCP
Professor of Diabetes and Autoimmunity/Consultant Physician,
Department of Diabetes and Metabolism, St Bartholomew's and
Royal London School of Medicine, London, UK

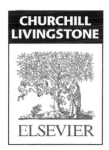

CHURCHILL
LIVINGSTONE

ELSEVIER

EDINBURGH   LONDON   NEW YORK   OXFORD   PHILADELPHIA   ST LOUIS   SYDNEY   TORONTO   2006

CHURCHILL LIVINGSTONE
ELSEVIER

First published 2005

ISBN 0443073031

British Library Cataloguing in Publication Data
A catalogue record for this book is available from the British Library

Library of Congress Cataloging in Publication Data
A catalog record for this book is available from the Library of Congress

---

Note

Knowledge and best practice in this field are constantly changing. As new research and experience broaden our knowledge, changes in practice, treatment and drug therapy may become necessary or appropriate. Readers are advised to check the most current information provided (i) on procedures featured or (ii) by the manufacturer of each product to be administered, to verify the recommended dose or formula, the method and duration of administration, and contraindications. It is the responsibility of the practitioner, relying on their own experience and knowledge of the patient, to make diagnoses, to determine dosages and the best treatment for each individual patient, and to take all appropriate safety precautions. To the fullest extent of the law, neither the Publisher nor the Authors assumes any liability for any injury and/or damage to persons or property arising out of or related to any use of the material contained in this book.

The Publisher

The publisher's policy is to use **paper manufactured from sustainable forests**

Printed in China

Preface

The aim of this book is to provide the cardinal features and descriptions of endocrine diseases and diabetes mellitus. The relevant physiology and anatomy have been included since these guide the understanding of tests and management. Where possible, summaries of crucial trials and a full range of management options are provided. The role of more specialised investigations, such as dynamic endocrine tests and magnetic resonance imaging, are discussed. Although some of the conditions described in the book are rarely seen, their clinical significance is high because many are treatable. The text is mainly intended for senior medical students, endocrinologists in training and general medical practitioners. It should provide sufficient detail for preparation for postgraduate general internal medicine examinations such as the MRCP(UK).

S.L.C
D.L.

Acknowledgements

The authors are very grateful to patients for allowing their images to be used in this book. We are very grateful to our colleagues who provided clinical expertise or images: Mr Fary Afshar (Consultant Neurosurgeon); Mr John Yeh (Consultant Neurosurgeon); Professor Rodney Reznek (Consultant Radiologist); Dr Jane Evanson (Consultant Radiologist); Dr Alison McLean (Consultant Radiologist); Professor Keith Britton (Consultant Nuclear Medicine); Dr Nick Plowman (Consultant Radiotherapist); Mr Robert Carpenter (Consultant Surgeon); Dr Dan Berney (Consultant Pathologist); Dr Les Perry, Dr Kate Noonen and Professor Jacky Burrin (Biochemistry); Dr Emma Spurrell (CRUK Fellow); the Endocrine nursing team on Garrod/ Francis Fraser, St Bartholomew's Hospital, London; and the Diabetes team, including Mohammed Al-Bader, Binu Varghese and Antonietta Gigante. We are very grateful to the editors and illustrators at Elsevier for their expert help.

Contents

General endocrinology

Introduction

Definitions: hormones and feedback

Endocrinology is based on the two fundamental principles: the action of hormones and regulation by feedback loops. A hormone is defined as a chemical messenger made by tissues or ductless glands and secreted directly into the blood. (Hormone is from the Greek *hormao* (to arouse or to excite).) Hormones circulate in the blood and have endocrine actions at many tissues. This basic definition may be extended to include hormones secreted from nerve endings, for example antidiuretic hormone (ADH; vasopressin). Some hormones also have *paracrine* actions, where effects occur on the same tissue as secretion, or *autocrine* actions, where effects are on the same cell that made the hormone. The feedback loop involves the effect a hormone has on its own tissue, usually to inhibit its own secretion and manufacture.

Types of hormone

There are three main categories of hormones: steroids, tyrosine (an amino acid) derivatives, such as thyroid hormones and catecholamines, and proteins (Fig. 1). Steroids and thyroid hormones are fat soluble and diffuse across the cell membrane to bind intracellular receptors in the cytoplasm or nucleus (Fig. 2). In order to maintain their solubility in an aqueous solution like blood, they must be attached to carrier proteins. In contrast, protein hormones and catecholamines are water soluble and do not diffuse across cellular membranes. They interact with cell surface receptors spanning the cell membrane, which signal via second messengers to the nucleus (Fig. 3). Many protein hormones have circulating binding proteins that regulate the availability of the hormone to its receptor. Hormones act in many ways on a tissue, changing intracellular signalling pathways and activating or repressing the expression of genes in the nucleus.

Regulation of hormones

The level of a hormone in plasma is tightly regulated, by feedback and other

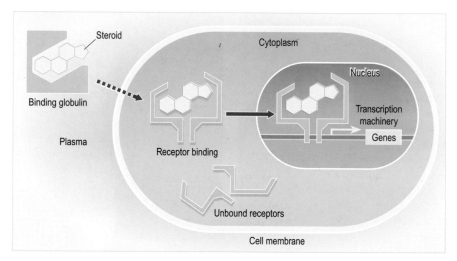

Fig. 2 **Lipid-soluble hormone signalling via intracellular receptors.** An example of this is cortisol.

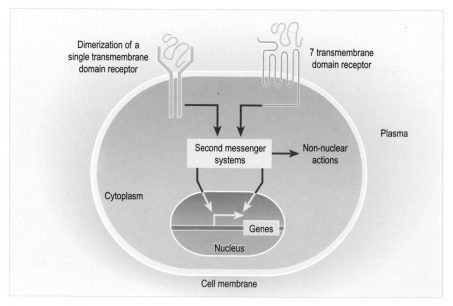

Fig. 3 **Peptide hormone action via membrane-bound receptors.**

Fig. 1 **Types of hormone.**

A steroid with 4 carbon rings

Thyroxine

A polypeptide hormone with cysteine bonds and a gycosylated side-chain (CHO)

Adrenaline (epinephrine)

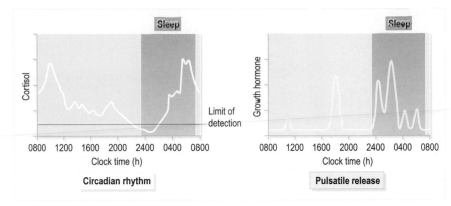

Fig. 4 **Comparison of the pattern of hormone levels in a 24-hour period for cortisol and growth hormone.**

influences. Many hormones have a circadian rhythm (from the Greek *circa* (about) and *dies* (a day)) to their release; for example cortisol has high levels in the early hours of the morning and low levels at midnight (Fig. 4). Hormones are also released in pulses, for example growth hormone, which is released in nocturnal bursts and is generally undetectable in the day (Fig. 4). The main determinant of the level of a hormone in the blood is the rate of release from stores in the endocrine gland. Hormones are maintained in a readily releasable pool within cells for rapid secretion. The rate of new synthesis of hormones is also efficiently regulated. Finally, the rate of metabolism or breakdown has a major influence on circulating hormone levels. Hormones are usually metabolized by the liver or kidney, but some are broken down in peripheral cells or in the plasma (Table 1). The circulating concentrations of many hormones are significantly affected by illness, stress or drugs (Table 2). Therefore, the interpretation of plasma hormone levels is very dependent on the conditions under which a sample is taken. In general, normal ranges for hormones relate to a sample taken at 0900 h in an unstressed healthy adult.

Table 2 **Non-physiological controls on circulating hormone levels**

Hormone	Control
Inhibition	
Thyroid hormones	Physical illness, benzodiazepine drugs
Gonadotrophins	Steroids, weight loss, exercise
Adrenocorticotrophic hormone	Corticosteroids
Stimulation	
Adrenocorticotrophin	Acute illness
Prolactin	Physical and mental stress, anti-emetic drugs, (dopamine receptor antagonists)

Measurement of hormones

Hormones are most commonly measured in serum or plasma using immunoassays. These assays depend on a specific antibody raised against a hormone. The specific antibody is chemically bound to a solid surface (often coated on the bottom of the wells of plastic plates). The serum or plasma is placed on the antibody-coated solid surface and specific binding occurs. The concentration of the hormone is then measured by one of two common methods: a single-site competitive assay; or, a two-site non-competitive assay (Fig. 5). The single-site assay immunoassay quantifies the number of

Fig. 5 **The general principles of immunoassay.**

unbound antibody sites. It is used for small molecules such as steroid hormones. The two-site assay uses a specific antibody targeting a second site on the bound hormone and is used for measuring large molecules such as polypeptide hormones. Accurate quantification is performed by plotting the signal from the patient sample against multiple standard samples containing known concentrations of the hormone. Common pitfalls of immunoassays are:

- lack of true specificity of some antibodies
- interference by anti-idiotype antibodies in the patient sample with the specific antibody
- interference by proteins or chemicals in the patient sample with the assay.

It should be routine to retest results that do not match the clinical situation in a different immunoassay.

Table 1 **Main organs metabolizing hormones**

Hormone	Organ
Prolactin	Kidney
Steroids	Kidney and liver
Thyroid hormones	Intracellular mechanisms
Catecholamines	Plasma

Hormones

- Hormones are chemical messengers.
- Lipid-soluble hormones diffuse into the cell.
- Water-soluble hormones bind cell surface receptors.
- Hormones can have endocrine, paracrine or autocrine actions.
- Feedback control is a major method of regulation of hormone levels.

The thyroid: basic concepts

Anatomy

The normal thyroid consists of pear-shaped left and right lobes (Fig. 1). The lobes extend from the thyroid cartilage to the 6th tracheal ring. The isthmus joins the anterior parts of the lobes and crosses the 2nd to 4th tracheal rings. The cricoid cartilage is an easy landmark to identify and the tracheal rings extend beneath this cartilage. Thyroid tissue is organized into follicles, which are lined by a single layer of epithelial cells and contain colloid (Fig. 2). The parafollicular or C-cells lie between the follicles. The thyroid develops from the 12th week of fetal life.

The normal thyroid gland is not visible or easily palpable. By the time a goitre is palpable, there has usually been a doubling of the size of the gland. Once a goitre is visible, it is about three times the size of a normal gland. The surface anatomy of the thyroid is of great importance for clinical evaluation. Note that if the trachea cannot be palpated, usually because of a cervical kyphosis, the thyroid gland will be retrosternal.

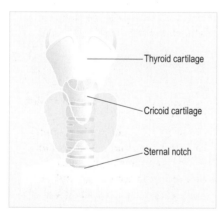

Fig. 1 **A diagram of normal thyroid surface anatomy.** The thyroid lobes and isthmus are in yellow. The thyroid and cricoid cartilages and sternal notch are indicated. The cricoid cartilage and tracheal rings lie inferior to the thyroid cartilage.

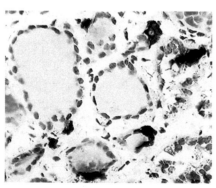

Fig. 2 **Histological section of a thyroid showing four thyroid follicles with C-cells (stained dark brown) in the parafollicular spaces.**

Thyroid hormone synthesis

The thyroid mainly produces thyroxine (T_4) and triiodothyronine (T_3). Both are derived from the amino acid tyrosine and iodine. Iodine is trapped in the epithelial cells of the thyroid gland via an active transport mechanism; it is then attached to tyrosine residues within a thyroid protein called thyroglobulin. This protein is secreted into the follicle to form a colloid (Fig. 3). Further enzyme reactions form T_4 and T_3 in thyroglobulin from which they can be secreted. Most normal thyroid secretion is in the form of T_4 (about 80 µg/day), with a small amount of T_3 (10 µg/day). The thyroid also secretes calcitonin, which is produced from the C-cells.

Thyroid hormone physiology

The main stimulation of thyroid hormone release and synthesis is thyroid-stimulating hormone (TSH) from the pituitary (Fig. 4). TSH acts through a surface receptor on the thyroid. TSH is under negative feedback at the level of the hypothalamus and pituitary, which sense the level of thyroid hormones in the plasma. Several non-thyroidal conditions can also change thyroid function:

- physical stress
- pregnancy
- drugs (Table 1)
- foods (e.g. containing iodine or flavones).

High levels of luteinizing hormone (LH) and human chorionic gonadotrophin

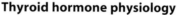

Table 1 **Some drugs that commonly affect thyroid function**	
Drug	**Effect**
Amiodarone	Increases iodine/causes thyroiditis
Glucocorticoids	Suppresses TSH
Oestrogens	Increases thyroid-binding globulin
Benzodiazepines	Suppresses TSH

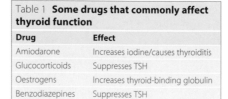

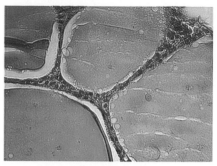

Fig. 3 **Normal thyroid histology.** The pink-stained smooth material in the follicles is colloid.

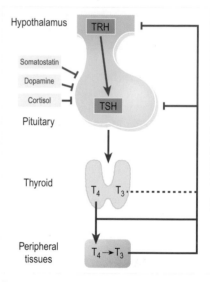

Fig. 4 **The hypothalamo–pituitary– thyroid axis.**

(HCG) can also stimulate the TSH receptor and increase thyroid hormone levels. In the blood, T_4 circulates bound to thyroid-binding globulin (TBG) and is converted in the peripheral tissues to T_3. Thyroid hormones pass into the cell and bind to nuclear receptors to regulate gene expression. Physiological actions of thyroid hormones include:

- cellular differentiation
- fetal development
- childhood growth
- mental function
- stimulation of metabolic pathways
- increased tissue oxygen consumption.

Thyroid tests

Serum TSH and free T_4 are reliable and convenient measures of thyroid function if they are measured in the same sample (Table 2). Measuring the serum TSH alone can be misleading because some patients with secondary

Table 2 **Tests for thyroid function**	
Test type	**Parameters measured**
Thyroid hormones	TSH, free T_4, total T_4, free/total T_3, sex hormone-binding globulin, thyroglobulin, thyroid antibodies
Radiology	Chest X-ray, thoracic inlet X-ray, thyroid ultrasound
Nuclear medicine	Technetium isotope, iodine isotope
Thyroid biopsy	Needle biopsy, thyroidectomy

hypothyroidism caused by pituitary disease will have TSH levels in the normal range. Total T_4 measurements include both the free and the TBG-bound hormone and will, therefore, be affected by the concentration of TBG. Several drugs, particularly oestrogens, may raise TBG concentrations and the total T_4, while the free T_4 will remain normal. Sex hormone-binding globulin (SHBG) is produced by the liver in response to thyroid hormones and may reflect the tissue effects of thyroid hormones. Serum thyroglobulin is a marker of the amount of differentiated thyroid tissue and is most useful in the follow-up of patients with thyroid carcinoma. Most laboratories will test for circulating antibodies against thyroid peroxidase or microsomes, and thyroglobulin, which are common in the general population. Radiology, isotope studies and biopsies are most useful in the investigation of goitres.

Thyroid and endocrine autoimmunity

Autoimmune disease is a common cause of thyroid pathology. The autoimmune pathogenesis is characterized by a lymphocytic infiltration in the thyroid (Fig. 1, p. 10) and serum antibodies against thyroid peroxidase, thyroglobulin, and thyroid-stimulating hormone receptor. About 5% of the UK population has circulating anti-thyroid antibodies. Autoimmunity may be classified into organ-specific and non-organ-specific. Patients with thyroid autoimmune disease are at increased risk of other autoimmune diseases, but particularly organ-specific conditions:

- vitamin B_{12} deficiency due to pernicious anaemia (gastric parietal cell and intrinsic factor antibodies)
- Addison's disease (adrenal antibodies)
- primary hypoparathyroidism.

The end result of the autoimmune process is fibrosis and atrophy of the gland and an irreversible failure of hormone production.

Iodine deficiency

Iodine deficiency is the commonest cause of thyroid disease worldwide. Iodine is lacking in the soil in mountainous regions and in inland areas. 30 % of the world population has been estimated to be iodine deficient. The clinical consequences of iodine deficiency are:

- abnormal thyroid function
- endemic goitre
- endemic cretinism
- perinatal death
- infant mortality
- infertility.

The commonest pathology is a goitre, which develops because of hyperplasia of thyroid tissue as an adaptation to low iodine levels. The most serious manifestation of iodine deficiency is endemic cretinism which classically includes mental retardation, with either severe hypothyroidism (myxoedematous cretinism), or neurological features such as deaf-mutism and gait disturbance (neurological cretinism). About 40 million people suffer mental handicap due to iodine deficiency and endemic cretinism affects over 10 million people.

Iodine intake can be measured by 24-hour urinary iodine excretion. The treatment of iodine deficiency is to increase iodine in the diet. Seafood contains high levels of iodine. In the UK, iodine is added to animal feed and good iodine levels are obtained from dairy products, meat and eggs. In endemic areas, use of sodium iodide table salt is beneficial. Conversely, excessive intake of iodine (for example, seaweed) in iodine-rich regions such as the UK can lead to thyrotoxicosis.

Examination of the thyroid

The basic assessment of the thyroid is the examination of the:

- Hands
- Eyes
- Neck
- Skin
- Pulse and heart.

The hand is examined for a tremor, nail changes, clubbing, sweating, heat or cold temperature. The eyes may show oedema or Graves' eye signs. The skin may show rashes or pre-tibial myxoedema (Fig. 5; p. 9). The neck is best examined from behind with the patient seated on a chair in the following order:

- Inspect for goitre
- Identify cricoid cartilage and sternal notch
- Gently palpate for tracheal deviation
- Palpate over trachea and under sternomastoid muscles for goitre
- Palpate for anterior and posterior triangle cervical lymph nodes
- Ask patient to swallow (supply a glass of water) while feeling a mass to check it rises
- Listen to a mass with a stethoscope.

The thyroid

- The thyroid covers the upper tracheal rings.
- Pituitary TSH stimulates thyroid hormone production/secretion.
- Both T_4 and T_3 are derived from iodinated tyrosine.
- The thyroid produces mostly (80%) T_4.
- The thyroid produces 80 µg T_4 per day.
- Most T_3 is formed from T_4 in peripheral tissues.
- Thyroid hormones affect all tissues/metabolic pathways.

Growths: goitres and cancer

Definition

A goitre is an enlarged thyroid gland (the term is derived from the Greek word for a shield).

The anatomy is discussed on p. 4.

Aetiology

Goitre can be caused in a number of ways:

- nodular goitre
- Graves' disease
- Hashimoto's thyroiditis
- iodine deficiency
- thyroid neoplasia
- goitrogens
- radiation exposure
- deposition diseases (amyloid).

The commonest causes of goitre in the Western world are nodular thyroid disease and autoimmune disease. Nodular thyroid disease develops because of focal hyperplasia of thyroid follicular cells, in combination with scaring and other damage to the connective tissue network of the thyroid. A degree of subclinical thyroid nodularity is very common over the age of 40 years. Graves' disease stimulates diffuse enlargement of the thyroid follicles through the presence of thyroid-stimulating immunoglobulins. In Hashimoto's thyroiditis, a lymphocytic infiltration causes thyroid swelling. Iodine deficiency is the commonest cause of goitre world-wide and it has been suggested that at least 650 million people suffer goitre from iodine deficiency.

Symptoms and signs

Nodular goitre

The presenting symptoms of a nodular goitre include

- slow development of lump in neck
- insidious onset of thyrotoxicosis

- dysphagia
- cough
- sudden goitre enlargement
- sudden neck pain
- stridor
- hoarse voice (rare, suggests carcinoma).

The onset of a nodular goitre is commonly insidious, with a gradual increase in the number of nodules. The nodules are almost always firm, move freely with swallowing and are non-tender (Fig. 1). Patients may have symptoms of hyperthyroidism. However, in contrast to the hyperthyroidism of Graves' disease, the oversecretion of thyroid hormones develops insidiously. An incidental finding of tracheal deviation on a chest radiograph is a common presentation of a goitre (Fig. 2). An unusual acute presentation may be caused by haemorrhage into a degenerating nodule or cyst. All acute presentations require urgent assessment and intervention because of the risk to the airway. A single nodule raises the question of thyroid neoplasia. Similarly, a particularly large or dominant nodule in a gland with multiple nodules carries a risk of carcinoma of approximately 10%.

Autoimmune thyroid disease

Patients with autoimmune goitres may present with symptoms and signs of thyrotoxicosis (Graves' disease) or hypothyroidism (Hashimoto's disease). The onset of symptoms is often acute and the goitre may be an incidental finding on examination. However, a significant minority of patients with autoimmune thyroid disease may be

euthyroid. The neck swellings are usually diffuse, firm and symmetrical. However, in severe or long-standing Graves' disease, irregular hyperplasia, degeneration and metaplasia occur in the gland and nodules may develop. Therefore, thyroid nodules do not exclude a diagnosis of Graves' disease. A bruit may be heard in patients with Graves' thyrotoxicosis. Tracheal deviation is unusual and symptoms and signs of compression of neck structures are rare.

Investigations

Measurement of serum TSH and free T_4 are essential. Furthermore, a T_3 level should be tested in anyone with a suppressed TSH. A chest and thoracic inlet radiograph will help to reveal the retrosternal extension and tracheal deviation or narrowing. X-rays will also reveal calcifications. Several pathologies are associated with thyroid calcification, including papillary and medullary thyroid cancers, but the commonest cause of calcification is old haemorrhages.

An ultrasound of the thyroid is an excellent test to confirm thyroid nodularity. Ultrasound will also give an accurate size of a nodule, the number of nodules and the presence of cystic lesions. A particularly large or dominant nodule can also be identified. The ultrasound scan is also a useful baseline for future tests to follow small (< 1 cm) lesions or small goitres. Computed tomographic scanning is helpful in evaluating large or retrosternal goitres (Fig. 3).

Technetium thyroid scanning (Fig. 4) is useful in identifying cold nodules (which may be carcinomas) and hot nodules (which are easily treated with radioiodine). Fine-needle biopsy of dominant, cold or hard nodules should yield diagnostic information in 80% of cases when performed by experienced physicians. Ultrasound-guided needle biopsy by an experienced radiologist is useful for drainage and diagnosis of thyroid cysts.

Important initial tests include:

- serum TSH, free T_4
- serum T_3 should always be checked if TSH is low
- thyroid peroxidase (or microsomal) autoantibodies
- thyroid ultrasound
- chest and thoracic inlet radiographs.

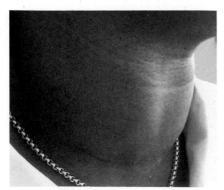

Fig. 1 **A moderately sized nodular goitre.**

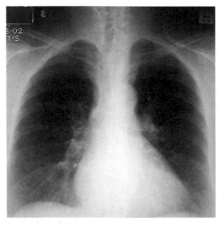

Fig. 2 **A chest radiograph showing deviation of the trachea to the right caused by a retrosternal goitre.**

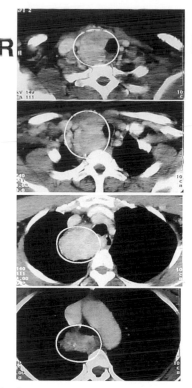

Fig. 3 **A right-sided nodular goitre (circled) with trachea shifted to the left.** The patient had had a left hemithyroidectomy at another hospital, but the right lobe continued to grow. The computed tomographic scan of the neck and chest shows the goitre in the neck (top image) extending through many cuts deep into the middle mediastinum (bottom image). A specialist endocrine surgeon managed to deliver this goitre into the neck without a sternal split and successfully removed it.

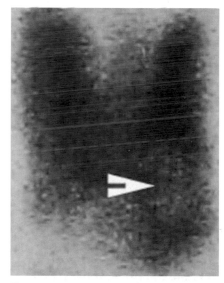

Fig. 4 **A technetium-uptake scan showing a cold nodule in the left lower pole.**

Management

Medical treatment
Thyroxine should only be used in patients with elevated TSH levels, and the aim should be to maintain the TSH level in the normal range. Treatment with thyroxine has been used to suppress TSH secretion. The rate of goitre size reduction on this treatment is poor. Furthermore, suppression of TSH puts the patient at risk of osteoporosis and atrial fibrillation in the long term.

Radioiodine
A sufficient dose of radioiodine will result in a 50% reduction in the size of non-toxic nodular goitres over a 2-year follow-up period. Radioiodine is safe (see Box 1, p. 9). Patients must be followed closely for radioiodine-induced hypothyroidism.

Surgery
Surgery remains a highly effective treatment in the hands of an expert surgeon. In nodular thyroid disease, recurrent nodules occur unless sufficient thyroid tissue is removed (Fig. 3). Therefore, a near-total thyroidectomy is recommended and patients will be dependent on lifelong T_4 replacement.

Thyroid cancer

Aetiology
The best documented risk factor for thyroid cancer is exposure to radiation. This may have occurred as a result of medical treatment (for example radiotherapy given for a childhood lymphoma) or radioiodine from nuclear fallout (as after the Chernobyl nuclear disaster in the Ukraine in 1986). Children under 14 years of age at the time of exposure are the most vulnerable. Rarely, thyroid cancer may be inherited. However, in most cases no aetiological factor for thyroid cancer is evident. Table 1 gives the main types and behaviours of thyroid cancer.

Symptoms and signs
The presentation is usually with a progressive swelling in the neck (Fig. 5), either because of the primary tumour or because of lymph node metastases. The patient is nearly always euthyroid. Nodules are usually either single and hard or are dominant nodules in a background of a nodular thyroid gland. Nodules in patients under 40 years of age should always be viewed

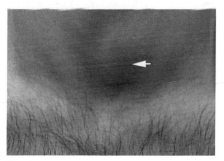

Fig. 5 **A follicular neoplasm presenting as a single nodule in a young male adult.**

as suspicious. Hoarseness of the voice may be a sign of recurrent laryngeal nerve compression or invasion; some tumours will be stuck down and infiltrate the surrounding tissue in the neck. Lymphadenopathy may be felt. There is a higher incidence of thyroid neoplasia in patients with Graves' disease and 10–20% of dominant cold nodules in multinodular goitres will be carcinomas. Therefore, a pre-existing thyroid diagnosis should not deter investigations for neoplasia. Distant metastases occur most commonly to the lungs or bones.

Management
Surgery is an essential part of the initial management of carcinoma of the thyroid and it is recommended that this be performed in the context of a specialist thyroid cancer programme. Thyroid cancer is usually very radiosensitive, so radioiodine an important treatment, initially to ablate the remaining normal thyroid, and subsequently used to target residual cancer. Life-long follow-up is required as recurrent disease may develop after many years. The prognosis is generally excellent with 10-year disease-free survival of over 90% in well-differentiated thyroid carcinoma.

Table 1 **Main types and behaviours of thyroid cancer**

Type	Behaviour
Papillary	Lymphatic spread
Follicular	Vascular spread
Huerthle	Histopathology not predictive of behaviour
Medullary	Associated with multiple endocrine neoplasia (MEN) II
Anaplastic	Very aggressive with local invasion; poor prognosis
Lymphoma	Associated with Hashimoto's thyroiditis

Goitres and cancer

- Goitres may be nodular or autoimmune.
- Goitres in the elderly are commonly retrosternal owing to kyphosis.
- Nodular goitres usually progress insidiously.
- Hard or fixed lesions or hoarseness suggest neoplasia.
- Check thyroid function and thyroid antibodies.
- Radiology: thoracic inlet and chest radiograph are useful as is thyroid ultrasound.
- Surgery is indicated for compressive symptoms.
- Radioiodine therapy will reduce gland size by 50% over 2-years.

Hyperthyroidism

Basic concepts and aetiology

Hyperthyroidism is defined as overfunction of the thyroid gland and is associated with a clinical state of thyrotoxicosis. The causes include

- Graves' disease
- toxic nodular goitre
- destructive thyroiditis
- iodine excess (Jod–Basedow effect)
- amiodarone
- TSHoma.

Graves' disease and nodular goitres are the most common causes. Thyrotoxicosis may occur without hyperthyroidism, most commonly in patients taking excessive thyroxine.

Symptoms and signs

Symptoms

The cardinal symptoms of thyrotoxicosis are:

- weight loss despite good appetite
- heat intolerance
- sweating
- palpitations
- agitation
- emotional lability
- poor concentration/memory
- diarrhoea
- pruritis
- muscle weakness
- oligomenorrhoea.

In Graves' disease, the symptoms often have a quick onset with a rapid progression and may be very severe. By contrast, the onset of thyrotoxicosis is often insidious in patients with nodular goitres. Symptoms may affect many organs because thyroid hormones affect every tissue and metabolic pathway.

Signs

The signs of thyrotoxicosis are:

- hot sweaty hands
- fine tremor
- agitation
- goitre
- resting tachycardia (> 80 beats/min)
- bounding pulse and wide pulse pressure
- atrial fibrillation
- high-output cardiac failure
- lid retraction
- gynaecomastia
- muscle weakness and wasting.

Serious signs are atrial fibrillation and fever. Patients with atrial fibrillation are at risk of embolism. Fever, confusion and dehydration are cardinal signs of

thyroid storm, an endocrine emergency. Thyroid storm may be iatrogenic, for example during or after thyroid surgery in a poorly controlled patient.

Investigations

The TSH level is suppressed and usually undetectable owing to feedback suppression by increased levels of T_4 and/or T_3. The sex hormone-binding globulin (SHBG) is often elevated.

Graves' disease

Aetiology

Graves' disease is classically a triad of autoimmune thyrotoxicosis, eye disease and pretibial myxoedema. It is associated with the presence of thyroid-stimulating immunoglobulins in the serum. The condition is probably partly inherited and is associated with other autoimmune conditions (Fig. 1). It is associated with autoimmune stimulation of fibroblasts and inflammatory cells. This affects the retro-orbital space (ophthalmopathy), skin (dermopathy) and fingers (acropachy). The non-thyroidal manifestations usually present close to the time of thyrotoxicosis, but occasionally may substantially pre- or postdate the thyroid problem. Radioiodine treatment and smoking are risk factors for worse eye disease.

Signs and symptoms

Many of the general signs of Graves' thyrotoxicosis are the same as in any cause of hyperthyroidism. However, the goitre of Graves' disease is usually diffuse, firm and smooth, rather than nodular. The presence of a bruit over a thyroid supports a diagnosis of Graves' disease.

Symptoms

The symptoms of Graves' ophthalmopathy usually relate to the extent of retro-orbital inflammation:

- pain behind the eye
- excessive tearfulness

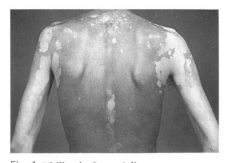

Fig. 1 **Vitiligo in Graves' disease.**

- grittiness and redness of the sclera (from exposure)
- double vision (diplopia caused by involvement of external ocular muscles)
- reduced visual acuity (compression of optic nerve)
- loss of colour vision (compression of optic nerve).

Signs

The commonest peripheral sign is retraction of the upper lid (Fig. 2). Retro-orbital inflammation may affect both the ocular muscles and the fat tissue (Fig. 3). Failure to close the eye may lead to exposure of the sclera and cornea (Fig. 4). The inferior rectus muscle is commonly affected, resulting in diplopia on upward gaze. When inflammation

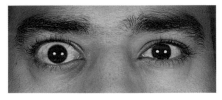

Fig. 2 **Retraction of the upper lid caused by unilateral exophthalmos on the right side.**

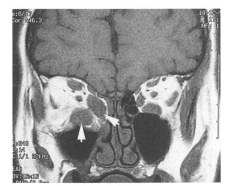

Fig. 3 **Magnetic resonance scan of the orbits in severe Graves' eye disease.** Severe inflammation and enlargement of the medial and inferior rectus muscles of the right eye are shown by the white arrows. Other orbital muscles in both eyes are also enlarged. There is a large amount of retro-orbital fat, especially on the right side, which is shown as a white signal.

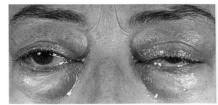

Fig. 4 **The patient is attempting to close her eyes.** There is exposure and inflammation of the sclera, particularly on the right, and excessive tear production.

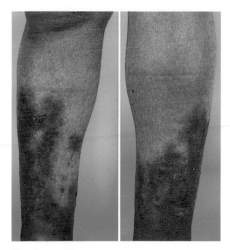

Fig. 5 **Pretibial myxoedema.**

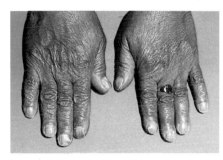

Fig. 6 **Thyroid acropachy, which is often associated with pretibial myxoedema.**

Table 1 **A suggested treatment regimen for severe Graves' thyrotoxicosis**	
	Details
Carbimazole	Once daily doses: 40 mg for 1 month, then 30 mg for 1 month, 20 mg for 1 month, and then 10 mg daily until reassessed
Propranolol	80 mg three times a day for 4 weeks
Written warning	Given for carbimazole agranulocytosis/rash
Full blood count	Check before starting therapy Give a FBC request form to patient in case of sore throat
Measurement of T_4 T_3 and TSH	Check at the end of each month's treatment

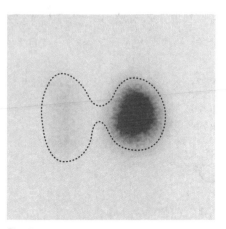

Fig. 7 **A technetium scan showing a hot nodule in the left lobe of the thyroid.**

Box 1 *Radioiodine therapy*

No increased risk of thyroid cancer in adults. There is a thyroid cancer risk to children under 14 years
Patients should stay away from young children for 14-21 days
Contraindications:

- Graves' eye disease,
- iodine allergy,
- neck compression,
- incontinence.

Thyroid function should be monitored starting after 8 weeks and then monthly for 6 months.

compresses the optic nerve, colour vision and acuity may be affected. Pretibial myxoedema classically affects the lower legs (Fig. 5). Nail changes and a form of clubbing (called thyroid acropachy) may occur (Fig. 6).

Investigations
Specific investigations include the measurement of thyroid peroxidase (or microsomal) antibodies, and autoantibodies to other organs (gastric parietal cells, liver/kidney microsomes, mitochondria, adrenal and antinuclear factor). The calcium, cortisol and vitamin B_{12} levels should be measured.

Treatment
Medical treatment with antithyroid drugs such as carbimazole is usually the first line of approach. A standard regimen is shown in Table 1. After a 12 to 18 month course, up to 50% of patients will be able to stop carbimazole and remain euthyroid. In any patient with thyrotoxicosis, the first month of treatment should also include propranolol (a β-adrenoceptor blocker) to control symptoms. Radioiodine and thyroidectomy are available for some indications, but in severe thyrotoxicosis adequate medical control before these treatments is essential, otherwise a

thyroid storm may be precipitated. The factors that predict a failure of remission after the 18 month course are a large goitre or male sex. In these cases, radioiodine may be used as a primary treatment provided the thyrotoxicosis is not severe.

Toxic nodular goitre

Aetiology
Thyroid nodules are common in those over the age of 40 years and occasionally develop autonomy, with a gradual and insidious progression to thyrotoxicosis. The condition is more often seen in the elderly.

Signs and symptoms
The main sign is a nodular goitre, which may be entirely retrosternal (see p. 7). Rarely patients may present with pain or sudden swelling caused by haemorrhage into a nodule.

Investigations
Initially, a suppressed TSH with normal T_3 and T_4 levels is found; later, frank elevation of T_3 and/or T_4 may develop. Quite frequently the diagnosis of nodular thyroid disease is made when the patient is re-examined in the light of a low TSH level on blood tests taken for other symptoms. Thyroid autoantibodies are usually negative. A chest X-ray and ultrasound scan may be needed to identify retrosternal extensions. Radioisotope scanning may show hot nodules (Fig. 7).

Treatment
Thyroid nodules usually progress and rarely resolve spontaneously. Therefore, remission from thyrotoxicosis is very unlikely, in contrast to Graves' disease. Life-long therapy is recommended. Radioiodine has the advantage of being safe and will reduce the size of the goitre (Box 1). Radioiodine is

contraindicated if there are signs of compression of structures in the neck or thoracic inlet. In these cases, near-total thyroidectomy after medical treatment is indicated. Medical treatment with carbimazole is effective at controlling hyperthyroidism but will not reverse the growth of nodules and will be required for life if this is the only treatment.

Hyperthyroidism

- Graves' disease and nodular goitres are common causes of thyrotoxicosis.
- Graves' disease is associated with skin and eye signs and other autoimmune diseases.
- Symptoms affect many organs.
- Atrial fibrillation and fever are signs of severe disease.
- Thyroid storm may be iatrogenic.
- Serum TSH is undetectable or suppressed.
- Antithyroid drugs, radioiodine and thyroidectomy are treatment options.

Hypothyroidism

Aetiology

Hypothyroidism is a clinical state caused by low T_4 levels, with an improvement of the symptoms and signs after adequate thyroid hormone replacement. The causes of hypothyroidism are classified into primary ($>95\%$) and secondary (Table 1). Primary hypothyroidism is very common, affecting between 5 and 20% of patients seeking medical attention. It is about three times more common in women and increases with age. The commonest cause is autoimmune thyroid disease, also known as Hashimoto's disease. A variety of antibodies to the thyroid may be detected in the circulation. Thyroid peroxidase (or microsomal) autoantibodies are most common and are predictive of thyroid failure. Other autoantibodies include those against thyroglobulin and antibodies that may block the TSH receptor. A combined autoantibody and T-cell-mediated attack causes inflammation and fibrosis in the thyroid. The histology shows a lymphocytic infiltration of the thyroid gland (Fig. 1).

Early in the disease, compensation for hypothyroidism is achieved by increased pituitary TSH secretion. Higher TSH stimulates more T_3 production from the thyroid and increases levels of the deiodinases that convert T_4 to T_3. This pituitary adaptation may preserve a euthyroid state (compensated subclinical hypothyroidism) for some months or years.

Table 1 **Causes of primary hypothyroidism**	
Common	**Rare**
Autoimmune lymphocytic	Infiltration
thyroiditis (Hashimoto)	Dysgenesis
Radioiodine	Thyroid hormone
Thyroid surgery	resistance
Drugs: antithyroid drugs	Iodine deficiency
(carbimazole), amiodarone,	Iodine excess
lithium	(Wolff–Chaikoff effect)

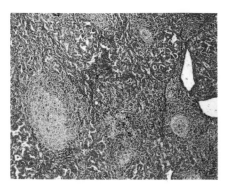

Fig. 1 Lymphocytic thyroid inflammation in Hashimoto's disease.

Symptoms and signs

Symptoms

The symptoms are hypothyroidism are:

- tiredness
- weight gain
- cold intolerance
- constipation
- dry skin
- tingling/pain in hands (carpal tunnel syndrome)
- hoarseness
- menorrhagia
- poor concentration/memory
- muscle pain or weakness
- swelling of face.

They vary enormously in severity and are non-specific. Symptoms usually start once the TSH is >10 mU/L.

Signs

The signs of hypothyroidism are:

- cold hands and skin
- slow pulse rate
- swelling of eyelids, face and limbs
- goitre
- slow-relaxing tendon reflexes
- apathy
- hair loss (capital and eyebrow)
- cerebellar signs
- carpal tunnel syndrome
- pericardial effusion.

The patient may look remarkably normal. In severe cases, a pseudo-dementia picture may predominate. In extreme hypothyroidism, there may be myxoedema coma.

Investigations

The investigations should aim to confirm the diagnosis of primary hypothyroidism, look for consequences of hypothyroidism and test for associated autoimmune diseases (Table 2). In primary hypothyroidism, the TSH is invariably raised. However, it is important to note that in secondary hypothyroidism, caused by pituitary or hypothalamic disease, the serum TSH may be normal or low (see p. 14). The practise of measuring TSH only, without a serum T_4 or T_3, may result in failure to diagnose pituitary or hypothalamic disease, because more than half the patients will have a TSH level in the normal range. If both free T_4 and TSH are normal, the patient is almost certainly euthyroid and an alternative cause for symptoms should be sought. Non-thyroidal illness may affect thyroid

Table 2 **Abnormal tests in primary hypothyroidism**	
Test	**Characteristics**
Full blood count	Normochromic anaemia
Urea and electrolytes	Low sodium
Liver function tests	Raised transaminases
Glucose	To exclude associated diabetes mellitus
Free T_4	Usually low
TSH	Always high
Cortisol	Low in associated Addison disease
Vitamin B_{12}	Low in associated pernicious anaemia
Autoantibody screen	To exclude associated autoimmune diseases
Electrocardiograph	To exclude occult heart diseases

function without symptoms and signs of tissue hypothyroidism (see p. 21).

Treatment

Most patients will be adequately treated with oral thyroxine. The daily dose is usually between 100 and 150 µg, best taken on waking. The treatment should be monitored with a serum TSH tested 6 weeks after starting thyroxine. Testing the TSH too early after starting thyroxine may lead to inappropriate increases in thyroxine dosage because the TSH takes time to return to the normal range.

There are several concomitant conditions that are potentially worsened by thyroxine therapy:

- heart disease: heart failure, infarction, angina
- chronic lung disease: breathlessness
- adrenal disease: hypoadrenal crisis.

Great care should be taken in those with heart disease because thyroxine increases the oxygen demand of most tissues as well as the myocardium. Starting thyroxine too rapidly has precipitated critical ischaemia, heart failure and myocardial infarction. Some patients may require hospitalization, cardiac monitoring and the slow introduction of low doses of thyroxine or liothyronine. Patients with subclinical adrenal disease may also become unwell as cortisol metabolism is increased.

Other thyroiditidies

Although Hashimoto's disease is the commonest cause of thyroid inflammation and dysfunction, several other clinical and pathological entities exist, some overlapping with

Table 3 **Thyroiditis**	
Disease/condition	**Characteristics**
Hashimoto	Lymphocytic thyroiditis (see above)
Graves	See p. 8
Postpartum	Painless lymphocytic thyroiditis with triphasic thyroid function
De Quervain	Painful inflammatory giant cell thyroiditis with high erythrocyte sedimentation rate
Riedel	Hard goitre, fibrosing thyroiditis, associated with midline fibrosis

Hashimoto's disease and conferring a risk of long-term hypothyroidism (Table 3). In the early stages of thyroiditis, the serum free T_4 may be high as a result of release of stores from a damaged gland (destructive thyrotoxicosis). Isotope thyroid uptake scans and Doppler ultrasound are useful in differentiating between a destructive thyroiditis and Graves' disease. A destructive thyroiditis shows no uptake on isotope thyroid scans, and hypoechogenicity and low to normal vascular flow on Doppler ultrasound.

Postpartum thyroiditis is a painless lymphocytic thyroiditis occurring in the first year after delivery. Autoimmunity may be stimulated by the presence of fetal cells in the maternal thyroid. Many patients have circulating thyroid peroxidase antibodies. The classic presentation is with an elevated serum free T_4 in the first 6 months after delivery, but patients are often clinically euthyroid or only mildly thyrotoxic (Fig. 2). In the second phase, usually 4–12 months after delivery, hypothyroidism occurs before recovery of normal thyroid function in the third phase. Nearly all patients will have recovered normal thyroid function by 12 months after delivery. Consequently, many patients can be observed rather than actively treated. However, in the long-term, hypothyroidism may develop in 50% and this condition should be

considered as part of the spectrum of autoimmune thyroid diseases. The main differential diagnosis is Graves' disease. An isotope uptake scan may help differentiation as this will show high uptake in Graves' disease and low uptake in thyroiditis. An isotope scan should not be performed in a patient who is breastfeeding.

Painful *subacute thyroiditis* (also known as *De Quervain thyroiditis*) is an inflammatory condition of unknown aetiology, although it is associated with upper respiratory tract infections. Tests for thyroid autoantibodies are usually negative and thyroid biopsy shows multinucleated giant cells rather than a lymphocytic infiltration. There is a painful swelling of the thyroid together with general symptoms such as fever, myalgia and fatigue. A destructive thyrotoxicosis characterized by a high serum free T_4 may be seen, but the condition is often subclinical. It is treated with aspirin or glucocorticoids. There is a risk of hypothyroidism in about 1 in 10 patients in the long term.

Thyroid disease and pregnancy

Pregnancy alters the physiology and biochemistry of the thyroid axis. Free T_4 levels usually remain in the normal range but tend to rise in the first trimester and fall in the last trimester. Thyroxine clearance increases and about half the patients with established hypothyroidism will need extra thyroxine. The serum TSH should be checked in each trimester and ideally should be 1–2 mU/L. A maternal goitre may be stimulated by pregnancy in iodine-deficient areas, but rarely in iodine-rich areas.

The maternal metabolic rate increases by 20% during pregnancy and the clinical signs of this may mimic

thyrotoxicosis. Human chorionic gonadotrophin (HCG) is produced by the placenta and stimulates the thyroid. When serum HCG levels are high, for example in multiple pregnancies, transient thyrotoxicosis may occur. Serum HCG peaks at about 10 weeks of gestation, after which HCG levels fall. Distinguishing HCG-related transient thyrotoxicosis from Graves' thyrotoxicosis may be difficult.

Autoimmune thyroid disease usually improves in pregnancy. In patients who have pre-existing Graves' disease, smaller doses of antithyroid drugs may be required. Thyrotoxicosis in pregnancy may be associated with fetal and neonatal thyrotoxicosis caused by transplacental transmission of thyroid-stimulating antibodies (Table 4). The fetal thyroid is capable of significant thyroid production after the 20th week of gestation. Treatment is essential as premature delivery, neonatal death and maternal cardiac failure are increased. The fetus should be monitored by ultrasound of the thyroid and recording of the fetal heart rate. A fetal heart rate of 180 beats/min indicates the need for urgent treatment. The main treatment is with antithyroid drugs that can cross the placenta. Propranolol may be needed in severe cases but is associated with growth retardation. Thyroidectomy should only be performed once the patient is euthyroid and radioiodine is contraindicated. At delivery, placental cord blood should be assayed to assess the neonatal thyroid state.

Table 4 **Transplacental transfer**	
Substances crossing placenta	**Substances that do not cross significantly**
Iodine	T_3 and T_4
Antithyroid drugs and propranolol	TSH
TRH	
Thyroid-stimulating antibodies	

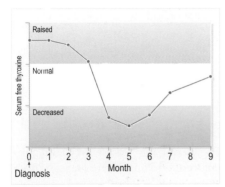

Fig. 2 **Triphasic thyroid function in postpartum thyroiditis.**

Hypothyroidism

- Hashimoto's thyroiditis is the main cause of hypothyroidism.
- Symptoms may affect many organs and are insidious.
- An important sign is slow relaxation of the tendon reflexes.
- Serum TSH is nearly always elevated.
- Wait 6 weeks before monitoring the effect of a change in the dose of thyroxine.
- Start thyroxine very carefully in patients with heart disease.

Pregnancy
- A painless lymphocytic thyroiditis can occur postpartum and last for up to a year.
- Patients with pre-existing hypothyroidism may need extra thyroxine.
- Autoimmune thyroid disease usually improves during pregnancy.
- Maternal thyrotoxicosis may be associated with fetal and neonatal thyrotoxicosis caused by transplacental transmission of thyroid-stimulating antibodies.

The pituitary: basic concepts

Anatomy and physiology

The pituitary gland lies at the base of the brain and is closely related to the chiasm of the optic nerves, the cavernous sinuses and the sphenoidal sinus (Fig. 1). The chiasm lies above the gland and can be compressed by large pituitary tumours. The cavernous sinuses are venous channels that lie on either side of the pituitary and each contains the carotid artery and the III, IV, ophthalmic division of the V, and VI cranial nerves. The sphenoidal sinus lies below and in front of the pituitary. The pituitary gland is contained in the pituitary fossa or sella turcica, a cup in the base of the sphenoidal bone. The pituitary fossa is covered by a layer of dura called the diaphragma sellae. The hypothalamus is connected to the pituitary by a stalk, which passes through a hole in the diaphragma sellae. The pituitary gland is split into two parts, the anterior and the posterior pituitary.

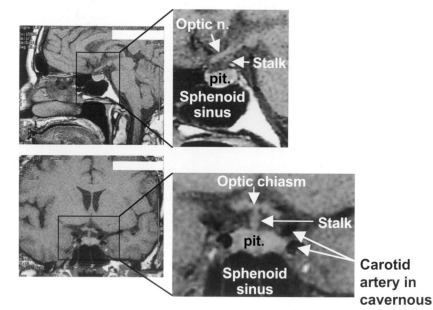

Fig. 1 **Magnetic resonance imaging shows the pituitary gland (pit.) and its relation to surrounding structures.** Top is a side (sagittal) view and below are frontal (coronal) views. n., nerve.

The anterior pituitary

The anterior pituitary produces at least six hormones under the control of hypothalamic factors that are transported to the pituitary via a portal circulation (Fig. 2A). A portal circulation is defined as flowing from one capillary network to another capillary network. Hypothalamic factors are released into capillaries in the hypothalamus. The portal circulation delivers these factors to capillaries in the anterior pituitary, where many of them stimulate the release and synthesis of anterior pituitary hormones. The exception is prolactin, which is inhibited by continual secretion (tonic inhibition) of the neurochemical dopamine. The production and release of hypothalamic and pituitary hormones are under negative feedback control (Fig. 2B).

The posterior pituitary

The posterior pituitary consists of nervous tissue. The nerve bodies have their origin in the hypothalamus and axons travel in the stalk to end at the posterior pituitary. Hormones, in particular antidiuretic hormone (ADH, vasopressin), are released directly from nerve terminals in the posterior pituitary into capillaries that drain to the circulation.

Symptoms and signs

Symptoms

The major symptoms of pituitary disease are listed in Table 1. The essential points to elicit are the function of key hormones, the presence of headache and visual failure.

Signs

The signs can be divided into those caused by oversecretion or lack of a hormone or neurological signs caused by compression by a pituitary mass. A comprehensive evaluation of the pituitary requires the ability to use an ophthalmoscope, assess visual acuity and to test the visual fields by confrontation (Fig. 3).

The classical signs in the eyes are bitemporal hemianopia, reduced visual acuity and pallor of the optic discs. The movement of the eyes should be tested for IIIrd, IVth and VIth nerve palsies. The general signs of pituitary hormone failure are outlined on p. 14. Signs of

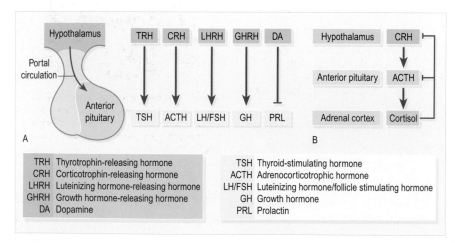

TRH	Thyrotrophin-releasing hormone
CRH	Corticotrophin-releasing hormone
LHRH	Luteinizing hormone-releasing hormone
GHRH	Growth hormone-releasing hormone
DA	Dopamine

TSH	Thyroid-stimulating hormone
ACTH	Adrenocorticotrophic hormone
LH/FSH	Luteinizing hormone/follicle stimulating hormone
GH	Growth hormone
PRL	Prolactin

Fig. 2 **The major hormones of the hypothalamus and anterior pituitary.** (A) Hypothalamic factors are transported in the portal blood supply and stimulate the release and synthesis of pituitary hormones. Dopamine is the exception in that it inhibits the release and synthesis of prolactin. (B) An example of negative feedback. Arrow indicates stimulation and bar indicates inhibition.

Table 1 **Major points in history-taking in suspected pituitary disease**

Type of effect	Results
Mass effects	Headache, visual problems, double vision
Oversecretion of hormones	Breast milk, poor libido, increase in shoe size, tight rings, easy bruising, muscle weakness, depression
Lack of hormones	Loss of periods, irregular periods, impotence, tiredness, nocturia, polyuria, thirst

hypopituitarism are often subtle and difficult to pick up unless the diagnosis is already known. The skin may be pale, fine and wrinkled and testes may be softer and smaller. It is much easier to identify signs of over-secretion of pituitary hormones, as in Cushing's disease (p. 28) or acromegaly (p. 18).

Investigations

In a non-specialist or emergency setting, several simple biochemical investigations can help to identify pituitary or hypothalamic disease. Basic pituitary function tests include:

- urine analysis and electrolytes
- renal function
- cortisol (at 0900 h)
- free thyroxine (T_4) and thyroid-stimulating hormone (TSH)
- prolactin
- oestradiol (women) or testosterone (men)
- Luteinizing hormone (LH)/follicle-stimulating hormone (FSH)
- Growth hormone (GH) and insulin-like growth factor-I (IGF-I)

Investigations include:

- magnetic resonance imaging (MRI) of pituitary/hypothalamus
- computed tomography (CT) of pituitary/hypothalamus if MRI is contraindicated (e.g. because of claustrophobia, metal implants or pacemakers)
- lateral skull X-ray: may show an expanded pituitary fossa.

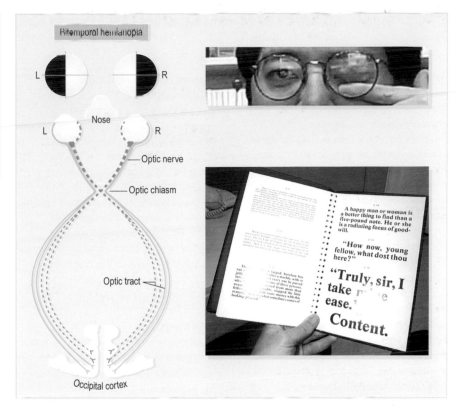

Fig. 3 **The anatomy of a bitemporal hemiopia.** The dotted line indicates the visual pathways disrupted by a pituitary tumour (yellow circle) compressing the optic chiasm. The light incident on the nasal side of the retina is not perceived (i.e. from the temporal field (shaded black)). The fields are easily assessed by the ability to see a red-coloured object as it is moved towards the centre of the field (top right) with the patient focusing on the examiner's eye. Visual acuity must be tested with a Snellen or J chart (the latter is shown bottom right).

Excellent images are obtained by MRI, which is safe, non-invasive and indicated in any patient where there is clinical or biochemical suspicion of pituitary or hypothalamic disease. CT scans are useful in patients unable to have MRI, where haemorrhage into a pituitary tumour is suspected or to search for calcium deposition in craniopharyngiomas. Where there is a waiting list for routine MRI and a large pituitary lesion is suspected, a lateral skull radiograph can be easily and rapidly performed and may show an enlarged pituitary fossa (Fig. 4). This finding would prompt an urgent request for MRI.

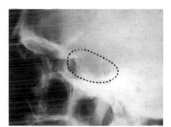

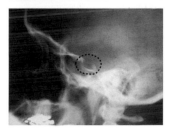

Fig. 4 **The pituitary fossa is seen in lateral skull radiographs from a large pituitary macroadenoma (top) and a microadenoma (bottom).** The dots outline the region of the fossa.

The pituitary

- The pituitary is connected to the hypothalamus by a stalk and receives a portal circulation from the hypothalamus.
- The anterior pituitary produces at least six hormones under the control of hypothalamic factors.
- The production and release of hypothalamic and pituitary hormones are under negative feedback control.
- Pituitary tumours cause mass effects, headache and visual disturbances, and effects of hormone inbalance.

Hypopituitarism and diabetes insipidus

Hypopituitarism is the failure of synthesis or release of pituitary hormones. Failure of the posterior pituitary results in diabetes insipidus. Anterior pituitary failure may be partial, as some hormone systems are more vulnerable to damage:

- growth hormone (GH): highly vulnerable
- gonadotrophins (LH and FSH): medium vulnerability
- adrenocorticotrophic hormone (ACTH; adrenocorticotrophin): medium vulnerability
- TSH: least vulnerable.

Isolated failure of individual anterior pituitary hormones is well recognized but rare. Pituitary failure developing in childhood may present as short stature (caused by GH deficiency) or pubertal delay (due to gonadotrophin deficiency).

Symptoms and signs

Symptoms and signs are often insidious, non-specific and reflect the wide effects of pituitary hormones (Fig. 1).

- tiredness
- loss of libido
- irregular periods
- loss of periods
- muscle weakness
- pallor
- hypotension
- nausea
- erectile dysfunction
- infertility
- central obesity
- fine wrinkling of the skin

Investigations

Basic pituitary function can be tested by blood taken at 0900 h and MRI of the pituitary and hypothalamus (see p. 13). In partial hypopituitarism, more complex tests are needed to assess GH and ACTH reserve. Serum insulin-like growth factor 1 (IGF-1) may be low in GH deficiency. GH and ACTH secretion may be stimulated by hypoglycaemia induced by controlled use of insulin (the insulin tolerance test). This test is contraindicated in patients with cerebrovascular or heart disease, fits, untreated hypoadrenalism, untreated hypothyroidism and hypokalemia.

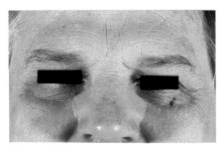

Fig. 1 **Fine wrinkles around the eyes, cheeks and forehead in a patient with pan-hypopituitarism caused by an anterior pituitary adenoma.**

Prognosis and treatment

Replacement therapy is available for every axis controlled by pituitary hormones (Table 1). All patients should carry extra supplies of replacement therapy and should wear a bracelet indicating their dependence on hormones (see p. 25). Patients with hypopituitarism are at increased risk of vascular diseases and treatment of cardiovascular risk factors such as hypercholesterolaemia, insulin resistance and diabetes mellitus are essential.

Diabetes insipidus

Physiology

The primary hormonal control of water excretion is via ADH (also known as arginine-vasopressin (AVP) in humans). This peptide hormone is synthesized in the hypothalamus by neurosecretory neurones and transported down the projections to be stored in granules at the axonal endings in the posterior pituitary (Fig. 2). ADH is released into the systemic circulation from the posterior pituitary and acts at the collecting duct in the kidney to

Table 1	**Treatments for hypopituitarism**
Deficiency	**Treatment**
GH	Recombinant GH
LH	Oestrogen or testosterone esters
FSH	Recombinant or purified gonadotrophins
ACTH	Hydrocortisone
TSH	Thyroxine

stimulate appearance of the water channel protein, *aquaporin-2*, on the surface of the cell. Water is then passively absorbed from the collecting duct through the water channel; the urine becomes concentrated and the plasma more dilute. The measure of concentration of solutes is *osmolality* (given as mOsm/L), which depends on the number of particles in solution and not on their size or weight. So plasma osmolality can be calculated from:

$$2 \times \text{sodium (mmol/L)} + \text{urea (mmol/L)} + \text{glucose (mmol/L)}$$

The primary physiological stimulus to ADH production is osmolality. ADH secretion is stimulated by a plasma osmolality above 280 mOsm/L (Fig. 3). Thus, within the physiological range, the urine osmolality is a reflection of

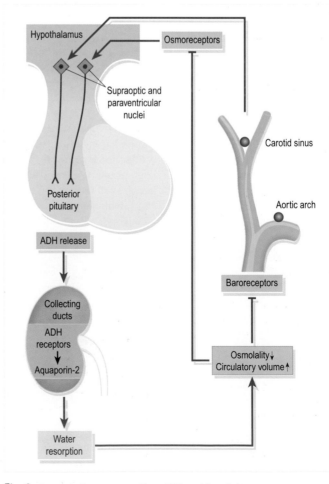

Fig. 2 **Control of water excretion.** ADH, antidiuretic hormone.

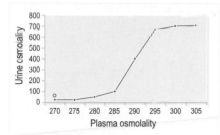

Fig. 3 **Increase of urine osmolality until a plateau is reached in response to increasing plasma osmolality (mOsm/L).**

plasma ADH concentration. Non-osmotic stimuli, for example hypotension, may bypass osmotic controls to increase ADH secretion.

Aetiology

The causes of diabetes insipidus may be classified into cranial or nephrogenic (Table 2). Note that anterior pituitary adenomas rarely cause diabetes insipidus.

Symptoms and signs

There are large volumes of dilute urine (polyuria), nocturia and thirst. The 24-hour urine volume is more than 2.5 litres, except in very mild cases. In severe diabetes insipidus, the 24-hour urine volume may reach 20 litres, and dehydration may be rapidly life threatening.

Investigations

In severe diabetes insipidus, the serum sodium and plasma osmolality are raised and the urine osmolality is inappropriately low. Normally, the urine osmolality is maximal when the plasma osmolality is 295 mOsm/L or above, and is at least twice the plasma value. Investigations include:
- plasma electrolytes and renal function
- plasma osmolality
- urine osmolality
- 24-hour urine volume
- water deprivation test (specialist use).
In mild or moderately severe cases, a high fluid intake may maintain the plasma osmolality in the normal range, and a water deprivation test will be needed to establish the diagnosis by

producing a concentrated plasma osmolality.

Treatment

The primary treatment is with desmopressin, an analogue of ADH. Desmopressin is available as a nasal spray, tablets or subcutaneous injection. Fluid treatment may also be needed. In mild or moderate cases, the conscious patient is able to compensate for water losses by drinking more. The main danger is if the patient cannot feel thirst (*adipsia*) or is unable to drink, for example in coma, and intravenous fluids may be needed. When treating severe dehydration, dextrose is preferred. Saline should be avoided because sodium retention may rapidly elevate the serum sodium.

Impaired water excretion

Impaired water excretion leads to hyponatraemia. The principle cause is non-osmotic ADH release; this can occur in
- hypotension
- cardiac failure
- dehydration
- diuretics
- liver failure
- porphyria.

In *pregnancy*, a physiological reduction in the threshold for ADH release lowers plasma osmolalities by 5–8 mOsm/L.

Inappropriate ectopic secretion of ADH (SIADH) occurs from small cell lung cancers and some other tumours; it is also associated with head injury and other cerebral pathologies. However, SIADH is quite rare and a clear set of criteria exist for its diagnosis:
- low plasma osmolality
- normal adrenal, renal and thyroid function
- urine osmolality not suppressed
- urine sodium > 20 mmol/L.

Symptoms and signs

Symptoms are non-specific and include headache, nausea, vomiting and unsteadiness. Seizures and coma occur with extremely low plasma osmolalities. Long-term sequelae, either of severe hyponatraemia or over-rapid correction, include neurological damage (classically central pontine myelinosis). A careful search should be made for volume depletion, and cardiac and liver disease.

Investigations

The serum sodium and plasma osmolality are low. Normally, the urine osmolality under such circumstances should be suppressed to < 100 mOsm/L, but in impaired water excretion will not be suppressed. The urine sodium is an important aid to diagnosis, since in volume depletion this is usually < 20 mmol/L owing to secondary hyperaldosteronism. Renal function, free T_4, TSH and cortisol at 0900 h should be tested. A chest X-ray is indicated. A CT or MRI of the brain may be indicated.

Treatment

In most cases of mild-to-moderate hyponatraemia, treatment of the underlying cause is sufficient to remedy the situation in a few days. Patients with dehydration will respond quickly to extra saline, although this should be under expert supervision and too rapid correction may be deleterious. In SIADH, fluid restriction usually improves the hyponatraemia while the underlying tumour is treated. ADH antagonists are in development and may be useful in this situation. Prevention is important; for example, intravenous dextrose solutions should be avoided in pregnancies, particularly when the patient is stressed by a second illness.

Table 2 **Causes of diabetes insipidus**	
Cranial	**Nephrogenic**
Idiopathic	Drugs: demeclocycline, lithium
After surgery or trauma	Hypokalaemia
Autoimmune	Hypercalcaemia
Neoplasms: germinomas, craniopharyngiomas	Genetic
Granulomas: sarcoidosis, Langerhans' cell histiocytosis, tuberculosis	Renal medullary diseases: analgesic nephropathy, sickle cell anaemia
Meningitis/encephalitis	Multiple myeloma
Vascular/infarction	
Genetic	

Hypopituitarism and diabetes insipidus

- Hypopituitarism is the failure of synthesis or release of pituitary hormones.
- Anterior pituitary failure may be partial, as some hormone systems (e.g. GH) are more vulnerable to damage. Failure of the posterior pituitary results in diabetes insipidus.
- Symptoms and signs are often insidious and non-specific.
- Life-long replacement therapy is needed.

Diabetes insipidus
- May be cranial or nephrogenic.
- Symptoms are polyuria and thirst.
- Plasma osmolality is raised and urine osmolality is inappropriately low.
- Treatment of cranial diabetes insipidus is with desmopressin.

Impaired water excretion
- Leads to hyponatraemia.
- Hypotension, dehydration and diuretics are common causes.
- Symptoms are non-specific.
- Urine osmolality is inappropriately high.

Non-functioning pituitary and hypothalamic tumours

Aetiology

The commonest lesion is a *benign adenoma* of the anterior pituitary, which represents about 10% of all intracranial neoplasms. Asymptomatic anterior pituitary adenomas are very common, and microadenomas are found in about 20% of autopsy cases. Microadenomas are less than 10 mm in maximum diameter, while macroadenomas are larger than 10 mm (Fig. 1). Adenomas are usually solid and vascular but may infarct or bleed (Fig. 2), or undergo cystic degeneration. Infarction of a pituitary adenoma may result in an empty but expanded pituitary fossa. Cystic masses of the pituitary are most commonly caused by cystic degeneration of a pituitary adenoma but may be *craniopharyngiomas* (a neoplasm with cystic and solid components, including dense areas of calcium deposition) or *Rathke's cysts* (non-neoplastic remnants of Rathke's pouch). Rathke's pouch is an embryological structure ultimately developing into the anterior and posterior pituitary.

Other tumours are less common (Table 1) and there is usually an

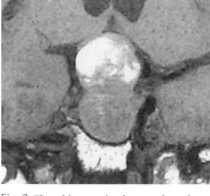

Fig. 2 **The white area is a haemorrhage into a large pituitary macroadenoma.**

indication from the clinical, biochemical or radiological picture that a mass is something other than an anterior pituitary adenoma. For example, diabetes insipidus is very rare with anterior pituitary adenomas but common in other diseases. Non-neoplastic masses are uncommon but rarely may represent part of a more systemic disease (for example, tuberculosis). Often, a diagnosis can only be made after surgical biopsy. Before surgery, care should be taken to exclude vascular lesions (such as carotid artery aneurysms; Fig. 3), prolactinomas and germ cell tumours. The last two diseases are usually not treated surgically.

MRI can usually distinguish between tumours arising from the suprasellar (above the pituitary) or parasellar (around the pituitary: cavernous sinus, sphenoid bone) regions and these lesions are much less likely to be pituitary adenomas.

Symptoms and signs

Pituitary tumours may present without specific symptoms and may be an incidental finding on a scan performed for non-specific symptoms. Symptoms may be classified into those resulting from a mass effect or from hypopituitarism (see p. 14). Symptoms

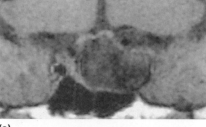

(a)

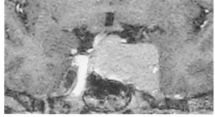

(b)

Fig. 3 **An aneurysm of the left carotid artery in the cavernous sinus filled the pituitary fossa.** (a) A magnetic resonance image without contrast showed a lesion that could be confused with a cyst. (b) This enhanced strongly when contrast was administered and indicated the vascular nature of the lesion.

and signs of non-functioning pituitary mass include:

- headache
- worsening visual acuity
- loss of visual field
- double vision
- bitemporal hemianopia
- other visual field defects
- reduced visual acuity
- loss of colour vision
- symptoms of hypopituitarism.

Symptoms and signs of non-functioning hypothalamic mass include:

- headache and visual disturbance
- polyuria (diabetes inspidus)
- loss of thirst sensation
- obesity and hyperphagia
- increased drowsiness
- precocious puberty
- body temperature abnormalities
- signs of hypopituitarism.

Headaches may be worse on waking, or if bending over or coughing. The pain may be localized to the forehead or be situated around one eye (caused by pressure on the ophthalmic division of the trigeminal nerve in cavernous sinus), or at the base of the occiput (referred pain from the posterior fossa caused by pressure on the clivus).

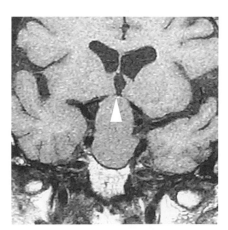

Fig. 1 **A pituitary magnetic resonance scan showing a coronal slice of a large pituitary macroadenoma.** The tumour arises from the sella and extends into the suprasellar region, compressing the optic chiasm (white arrowhead).

Table 1 **Masses of the pituitary or hypothalamus**	
Neoplastic	**Non-neoplastic**
Anterior pituitary adenoma	Tuberculosis
Craniopharyngioma and Rathke's cyst	Sarcoidosis
Other cranial neoplasms (e.g. meningioma, glioma)	Aneurysms and vascular lesions
Metastases (e.g. from breast or lung carcinoma)	Lymphocytic hypophysitis
	Langerhan's histiocytosis

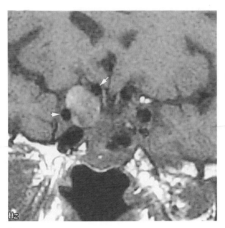

Fig. 4 **A recurrent pituitary adenoma in the right cavernous sinus.** The tumour invaded between the bend in the right carotid artery (indicated by two small white arrows) and caused palsy of the right cranial nerve III.

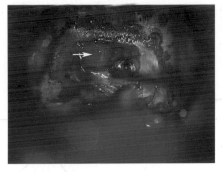

Fig. 6 **Operative view of hypophysectomy from the sphenoidal sinus. The metal curette has removed the tumour from the left side, leaving normal pituitary on the right (arrowed).** (Courtesy of Mr Fary Afshar.)

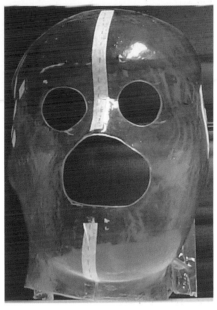

Fig. 7 **Plastic moulded mask used to fix the trajectory of radiotherapy beams in conventional three-field fractionated techniques used for pituitary tumours.**

Visual symptoms are also common. Hypothalamic tumours may present with symptoms caused by compression of hypothalamic nuclei.

A classical sign is a bitemporal hemianopia (see p. 13, Figure 3). Other patterns of visual field loss occur. Tumours in the cavernous sinus may cause palsies of cranial nerves III, IV and VI (Fig. 4).

Treatment of pituitary adenomas

Most patients will require surgical treatment, usually via a transsphenoidal approach (Figs 5 and 6). The main hazards of transsphenoidal hypophysectomy are further loss of pituitary hormones and leak of cerebrospinal fluid into the sphenoidal sinus; other hazards include:

- diabetes insipidus, usually temporary
- meningitis
- haemorrhage.

Precautions to reduce potential problems include:
- monitor blood pressure and urine output during and after surgery
- test serum cortisol 24 hours after stopping glucocorticoids
- reassess anterior pituitary function within weeks of operation
- give glucocorticoids to reduce postoperative oedema for several days after surgery for large masses compressing the optic nerve or hypothalamus
- prophylactic perioperative antibiotics are often used.

Pituitary radiotherapy is often considered after surgical removal of pituitary macroadenomas (Fig. 7). This reduces the 10-year recurrence rate from 50–80% to less than 5%. The convention is to give small daily doses via three beams to prevent toxicity to normal structures within the radiation field. Newer forms of highly focused radiotherapy (gamma knife) may be used to give a single high dose to recurrent or persistent tumours, provided the mass is sufficiently far from the optic chiasm and nerves. Box 1 outlines an approach in management of a pituitary or hypothalamic mass.

> ### Box 1 Practical approach to a pituitary or hypothalamic mass
>
> - Clinical evaluation for acromegaly and Cushing's disease.
> - Assess urine volumes.
> - Record visual acuity and fields.
> - Exclude medically treatable diseases (serum prolactin, human chorionic gonadotrophin).
> - Test for diabetes insipidus (plasma and urine osmolality).
> - Test for hypopituitarism (serum cortisol, free thyroxine, testosterone or oestradiol).
> - Chest X-ray.
> - Start treatment with hydrocortisone if deficient.
> - MRI scan of pituitary and hypothalamus.
> - Referral to a specialist centre.

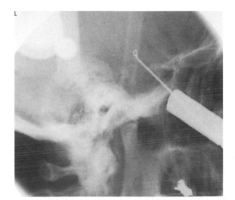

Fig. 5 **Transsphenoidal hypophysectomy.** The position of the surgical instruments is monitored by radiology. Note the expanded sella and the approach through the nose and sphenoidal sinus.

> ### Non-functioning pituitary and hypothalamic tumours
>
> - The commonest lesion is a benign adenoma of the anterior pituitary, which is often asymptomatic.
> - Non-neoplastic masses can occur as part of a systemic disease.
> - Symptoms can result from a mass effect (such as bilateral hemianopia) or from hypopituitarism.
> - Treatment is usually surgery, often followed by radiotherapy.

Functioning pituitary tumours

The commonest functioning anterior pituitary adenomas secrete prolactin or GH, and some adenomas make several hormones. ACTH-secreting adenomas are considered under Cushing's syndrome (p. 28). Other (rare) functioning adenomas are a TSHoma (may cause goiter and thyrotoxicosis) and FSHoma (FSH is usually inactive).

Prolactinomas

Prolactin maybe transiently elevated in normal subjects as it is a stress hormone. Physiological hyperprolactinaemia occurs in pregnancy and breastfeeding. Any interference with dopamine inhibition, for example therapeutic use of a dopamine receptor antagonist such as metoclopramide, will cause a high prolactin production (Fig. 1). Antibodies may cause clumping of prolactin molecules in a complex called macroprolactin (note: this should not be confused with the term macro-prolactinoma). Macroprolactin interferes with prolactin assays, generating an artefactually high serum prolactin.

A problem in diagnosis is that any pituitary or hypothalamic lesion that blocks dopamine delivery to the normal anterior pituitary will be associated with an elevated prolactin, even if the tumour is non-functioning. Such lesions are known as pseudo-prolactinomas (Fig. 2), and the raised serum prolactin arises from the normal pituitary. If serum prolactin levels are very high, >6000 mU/L (300 ng/mL), then a tumour is almost certainly a true prolactinoma.

Symptoms and signs

The overproduction of prolactin inhibits gonadal function giving rise to:

- oligomenorrhoea
- amenorrhoea
- galactorrhoea
- infertility
- loss of libido
- erectile dysfunction
- osteoporosis.

The commonest presentation is with oligo- or amenorrhoea and galactorrhoea (clear or white nipple discharge). The main long-term risk is osteoporosis.

Investigations

The first step is to confirm persistent elevation of serum prolactin in two or three samples taken an hour apart. The history should exclude physiological and pharmacological hyperprolactinaemia. Patients with artefactual macroprolactin may be asymptomatic or have atypical symptoms. Patients with true hyperprolactinaemia will need pituitary MRI and basal anterior pituitary function tests (p. 13).

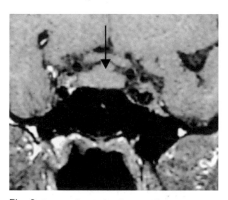

Fig. 2 **A pseudo-prolactinoma.** The tumour (arrowed) arose from the clivus bone behind the pituitary and blocked dopamine delivery to the normal anterior pituitary. The tumour was a chordoma.

Treatment

Prolactinomas are highly successfully treated with dopamine agonist drugs (bromocriptine or cabergoline) (Fig. 3). Some patients with side-effects on dopamine agonists (especially psychiatric reactions), or rare prolactinomas that fail to respond, may be treated by transsphenoidal hypophysectomy, radiotherapy or radiosurgery.

Management of infertility caused by a prolactinoma is highly successful (see p. 43). All patients should be monitored during pregnancy by clinical and visual field assessment. Pituitary MRI without gadolinium contrast may be safely used in pregnancy. The serum prolactin is of little value in monitoring prolactinomas in pregnancy.

Pseudo-prolactinomas do not shrink in size on treatment with a dopamine agonist, but note that there is a rapid fall of prolactin to undetectable levels (because the prolactin is secreted from normal anterior pituitary cells that are very sensitive to dopamine agonists).

Acromegaly

Oversecretion of GH by an anterior pituitary adenoma causes giantism before puberty and acromegaly after puberty. Giantism occurs because of active growth plates in the long bones before puberty. After puberty, the long bones do not grow further, but acromegaly causes growth of soft tissues, internal organs and some bones (Figs 4–6).

Symptoms and signs

The onset of symptoms and signs of acromegaly is often insidious, but progressive:

- growth of hands and feet
- tightening of rings
- wrist pain (carpal tunnel syndrome)

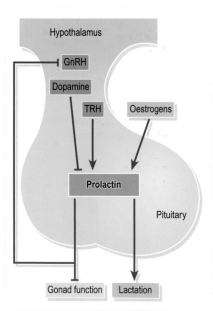

Fig. 1 **Physiological control of prolactin and its actions.** The arrows show stimulatory actions while bars show inhibitory actions. TRH, thyrotrophin-releasing hormone; GnRH, gonadotrophin-releasing hormone.

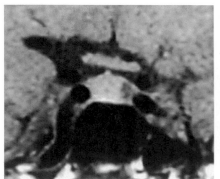 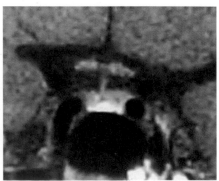

Fig. 3 **Resolution of a cystic microprolactinoma after a 2-year course of bromocriptine.**

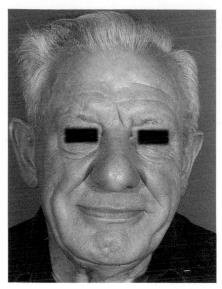

Fig. 4 **Coarsening of the face in acromegaly caused by growth of the frontal and mandibular bones and soft tissue swelling.**

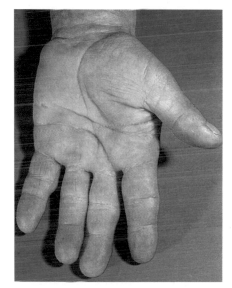

Fig. 5 **Enlargement of the soft tissues and bones of the hands results in a classical appearance of sausage-shaped fingers with thick doughy palms.**

- hand parathesiae (carpal tunnel syndrome)
- sweating
- dyspepsia
- erectile dysfunction
- menstrual irregularity
- hirsutism.

The signs are:
- large doughy hands
- sausage-shaped fingers
- advancement of lower teeth (prognathism)
- enlargement of tongue (macroglossia)
- separation of the teeth
- maxillary recession
- hypertension
- hyperinflated lungs
- carpel tunnel syndrome (usually bilateral).

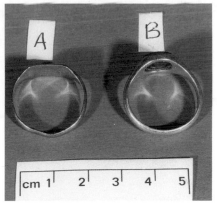

Fig. 6 **Enlargement of the ring size in a patient with acromegaly.**

The diagnosis is not infrequently made by someone who has not seen the patient for a number of years. Bilateral carpal tunnel syndrome (caused by swelling of the median nerve in the carpal tunnel) may result in presentation to an orthopaedic department. Patients have also been diagnosed by anaesthetists who have found intubation noticeably difficult because of the patient's large jaw and tongue.

Investigations

Most patients will have persistently raised serum GH levels. In normal subjects, GH release is pulsatile, but a profile of levels throughout a day will show some undetectable serum GH values. In acromegaly, serum GH levels remain persistently elevated in a day profile and they fail to suppress to undetectable levels after a 75 g oral glucose load. Serum IGF-1 levels are raised by GH stimulation of liver production (Fig. 7). An MRI of the pituitary will usually show the adenoma.

Treatment

The definitive treatment is transsphenoidal hypophysectomy. The likelihood of complete removal of the tumour and cure depends on the size of the adenoma and the preoperative GH levels. Larger tumours with high GH levels will be completely resected in only 40% of patients and will often require radiotherapy or medical treatment. The main option for medical treatment are somatostatin (Fig. 7) analogues.

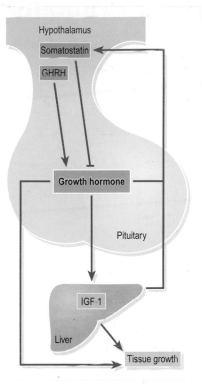

Fig. 7 **The growth hormone/insulin-like growth factor 1 (IGF-1) axis.** Somatostatin inhibition and GH-releasing hormone (GHRH) stimulation of GH release. GH and IGF-1 stimulate somatostatin production, resulting in a negative feedback loop.

Somatostatin analogues are available in monthly depot formulations (Somatuline Autogel or Sandostatin LAR). Such long-acting agents are cheaper and more convenient than octreotide (a short-acting analogue). Some patients respond well to oral dopamine-agonists. A GH receptor antagonist, somavert, is available for patients uncontrolled by other therapies.

Long-term complications
Long-term complications of acromegaly include:

- vascular disease
- hypertension
- diabetes mellitus
- sleep apnoea and chronic obstructive airway disease
- nodular goitre
- accelerated osteoarthritis
- hypercalciuria and renal stones
- colonic neoplasia.

Prolactinoma and acromegaly

- Prolactinomas cause galactorrhoea/amenorrhoea.
- Non-functioning tumours may mimic prolactinomas by blocking the control of prolactin release from normal lactotrophs.
- Prolactinomas are successfully treated medically with dopamine-agonists.
- Dopamine agonists may rarely cause psychiatric reactions.
- Acromegaly causes growth of soft tissues, internal organs and bones.
- Transsphenoidal surgery is the first-line treatment of acromegaly.
- Radiotherapy, somatostatin analogues and GH receptor antagonist may be needed.

Obesity and hypothalamic regulation of weight

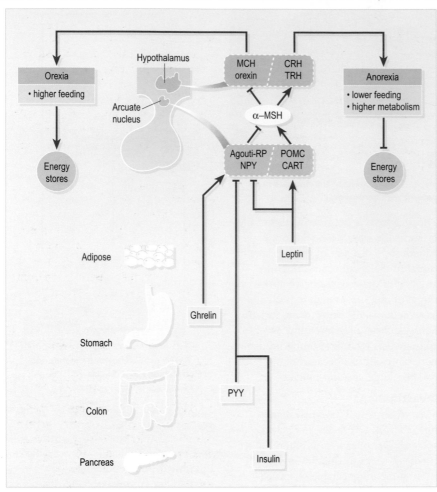

Fig. 1 **The regulatory network of feeding, hunger and satiety involves hormonal secretions from the hypothalamus, adipose tissue and gut.**

Table 1 **Measurement of obesity**	
Measure	**Value**
Body mass index^a (kg/m^2)	
Normal	20–25
Overweight	25–30
Obesity	> 30
Severe obesity	> 35
Very severe obesity	> 40
Abdominal obesity: waist diameter^b	
Obese male	> 102 cm (40 inches)
Obese female	> 88 cm (34 inches)

^{a}Given by weight (kg)/height^2 (m^2)
^{b}Measured mid-way between the lowest rib and the crest of the ileum with the patient standing with feet about 25 cm (10 inches) apart.

- hyperlipidaemia
- cardiovascular disease
- hypertension
- gallstones
- gout
- hypogonadotrophic hypogonadism
- osteoarthritis
- some cancers (mild increased risk).

A pharmacological approach to obesity may be indicated because of these associated risks (Table 2). Metformin should be interrupted for 48 hours before and after intravenous iodinated contrast media or during any severe illness. The occurrence of lactic acidosis and impairment of vitamin B$_{12}$ absorption are rare and largely theoretical risks; however, metformin should not be used if the serum creatinine is > 130 µmol/L. Gastric banding or bypass may be indicated for very severe obesity.

Table 2 **Drugs in obesity**	
Drug	**Comment**
Appetite suppressants	Side-effects include right-sided heart valve lesions, hypertension, tachycardia; latest version is sibutramine
Pancreatic lipase inhibitors	Prevent fat absorption from the gut and give fatty stools; a recurrence of weight gain can occur despite 2 years of treatment with orlistat
Insulin-sensitizing drugs	Metformin is associated with weight loss; reduces risks of progression to diabetes mellitus and vascular diseases. Metformin should be started at a low dose of 250 mg once daily to avoid gastrointestinal side-effects and should be slowly increased to a dose of 500 mg three times a day

> **Obesity**
>
> - Obesity is defined as excess body fat with a BMI > 30 kg/m^2.
> - The commonest cause is excess food intake (exogenous obesity).
> - Insulin resistance, hypothyroidism and Cushing's syndrome should be considered as potential causes.
> - The main risk is type 2 diabetes mellitus.
> - Diet and exercise programmes are essential treatment.
> - Metformin and orlistat may be useful drug treatments.

Obesity is defined as an excess of body fat. Obesity caused by excess food intake (primary exogenous obesity) has increased world-wide and an estimated 64% of Americans are now overweight or obese. This has resulted in an epidemic of type 2 diabetes mellitus. About two-thirds of type 2 diabetes mellitus in the USA is obesity related. Although much less common than primary exogenous obesity, endocrine causes of obesity are clinically very significant as they require specific treatment. Abnormalities of glucose metabolism and insulin resistance may precede obesity and invariably precede subsequent diabetes type 2 mellitus (p. 62).

The regulatory pathways for hunger and satiety involve a network of hypothalamic hormones, with influences from hormones secreted by adipose tissue and the gastrointestinal system (Fig. 1).

Clinical assessment

The severity of weight disorder can be assessed by several parameters (Table 1). Thick skin and acanthosis nigricans (see p. 40, Fig. 2) are features of insulin resistance. Clinical examination and investigations should screen for hypothyroidism and Cushing's syndrome. In view of the clinical significance of the diagnosis, a full evaluation is probably indicated even if only some features of Cushing's syndrome are present. Genetic causes of obesity present with extreme obesity from early childhood, developmental delay and characteristic physical, skeletal and facial signs (e.g. Prader–Willi syndrome: small hands, doe-like eyes). Hypothalamic damage and tumours may cause severe obesity. Many patients with hypothalamic damage will have disordered water balance (usually diabetes insipidus) or thirst impairment.

Management

Many patients have struggled with weight problems for years and have low self-esteem. A positive and encouraging approach is suggested and diet and exercise programmes should be strongly recommended. Many diet programmes are available, but a long-term reduction of calorie intake and a slow and progressive weight loss is the most rewarding goal. Exercise should aim to achieve at least 30 minutes of strenuous exercise three times a week. The complications of obesity include:

- diabetes mellitus
- sleep apnoea
- insulin resistance
- breathlessness

Non-endocrine illness and hormones

The hallmark of endocrine disruption caused by non-endocrine illnesses is that the hormonal abnormalities return to normal after treatment of the underlying illness. The commonest manifestation of severe systemic illness is the *sick euthyroid syndrome*. This is characterized by a fall in serum triiodothyronine (T_3) and, to some extent, serum T_4. The serum TSH usually remains normal but may decrease in severe illness. The serum thyroid hormone levels return to normal once the underlying condition is successfully treated. Thyroid hormone replacement is not recommended and does not improve the prognosis. Care should be taken to exclude secondary hypothyroidism (TSH deficiency) caused by pituitary–hypothalamic disease (p. 14).

Cardiorespiratory diseases

The commonest abnormality in cardiac failure is activation of the hormones regulating salt and water balance and vascular tone, giving rise to:

- secondary hyperaldosteronism
- increased catecholamines
- increased cortisol
- increased ADH
- increased atrial naturetic peptide.

These may exacerbate congestive cardiac failure by further salt and water retention and increasing peripheral vascular resistance. Serum cortisol levels are frequently high and should not be interpreted as Cushing's syndrome until re-evaluation after cardiac failure has been treated. Atrial arrhythmias are associated with polyuria caused by excess atrial naturetic peptide. In practice, the end result of these changes is commonly seen as hyponatraemia.

A common respiratory problem is sleep apnoea, which may elevate stress hormones such as catecholamines and cortisol. Furthermore, patients with sleep apnoea have hypertension and obesity and this may lead to the erroneous diagnosis of phaeochromocytoma or Cushing's syndrome.

Renal failure

Renal disease most commonly affects hormones regulating salt and water balance, calcium homeostasis, and red cell production. The endocrine consequences of renal failure are:

- low serum 1,25-hydroxyvitamin D
- elevated serum parathyroid hormone
- elevated plasma renin
- low serum erthyropoeitin
- elevated serum prolactin (reduced clearance)
- hypogonadism
- growth hormone resistance.

The kidney is the site of activation of vitamin D by 1-hydroxylation so renal failure is associated with deficiency of 1,25-hydroxyvitamin D. Sulphates and phosphates are not excreted efficiently in renal failure and this leads to binding of calcium and stimulation of parathyroid hormone secretion. The combination of hyperparathyroidism and 1,25-hydroxyvitamin D deficiency results in bone pain, tenderness, fractures and deformity. Many of these changes can be treated, for example with potent vitamin D analogues, leading to improvements in the clinical state and prognosis.

Liver failure

Haemochromatosis is a genetic disease of abnormal iron transport and storage, with abnormal liver function, skin pigmentation, impaired glucose tolerance and diabetes mellitus and hypogonadism. The hypogonadism is often a mixed type, with both testicular and gonadotrophin defects. The condition is exacerbated by alcohol use. Gynaecomastia is a typical clinical sign. In other causes of liver failure, endocrine abnormalities are common:

- gonadotrophin deficiency
- primary hypogonadism
- impaired clearance of androstenedione
- increased conversion to oestradiol
- raised serum sex hormone-binding globulin
- alcoholic pseudo-Cushing's syndrome
- raised TSH (reduced T_4 to T_3 conversion).

Oncology and paraneoplastic syndromes

Paraneoplastic syndromes are of clinical significance as they provide clues to the underlying diagnosis and they are a treatable cause of symptoms (Table 1). Clinical signs may be occult or atypical because the underlying neoplasm dominates the clinical picture. The diagnosis may be suggested by biochemical and haematological findings. Inappropriate ADH secretion may present with low serum sodium. Ectopic ACTH syndrome may not present with typical Cushing's syndrome, but instead there may be weight loss associated with high plasma glucose.

Table 1 **Paraneoplastic syndromes**	
	Neoplasm
Inappropriate ADH	Small cell lung cancer
Ectopic ACTH	Small cell lung cancer, carcinoid
Hypercalcaemia (parathyroid hormone-related peptide)	Squamous cell lung cancer, renal cell cancer, hepatoma and other gastrointestinal cancers
Erythropoietin	Renal cell cancer, haemangioblastoma

Endocrine disruption in non-endocrine illnesses

- Hormonal abnormalities return to normal after treatment of the underlying illness.
- Sick euthyroid syndrome is commonest manifestation of severe systemic illness.
- Cardiac and renal failure disrupt hormones regulating salt and water balance.
- Renal failure also causes hyperparathyroidism and deficiency of 1,25-hydroxyvitamin D.

Adrenal and endocrine hypertension: basic concepts

The adrenal glands produce hormones that are essential for the control of water and salt balance, and blood pressure. Adrenal hormones also affect sexual behaviour, reproductive function, carbohydrate metabolism and bone physiology. The adrenal gland is made up of two distinct endocrine systems, the cortex and medulla (Fig. 1). The cortex is a classical endocrine gland, making steroids under the influence of adrenocorticotrophic hormone (ACTH). The medulla is actually nervous tissue and is part of the sympathetic nervous system, secreting catecholamines, mainly adrenaline (epinephrine). There are some links between the cortex and medulla because cortisol acts at the medulla to induce the enzyme that converts noradrenaline (norepinephrine) to adrenaline.

Applied anatomy

The adrenal glands lie superiorly and anteriorly to the kidneys and are surrounded by the fat of the retroperitonium. The venous drainage from the right adrenal is via a short and wide adrenal vein, which drains directly and at right-angles into the inferior vena cava. Control of the right adrenal vein may be a challenging aspect of surgical resection of the adrenals. A tear in either the right adrenal vein or at the insertion into the inferior vena cava may cause serious retroperitoneal haemorrhage that is difficult to control. By contrast, the left adrenal vein drains at an angle into the left renal vein and is rarely difficult to control surgically. The main hazard of a left adrenalectomy is that the left adrenal lies close to the spleen

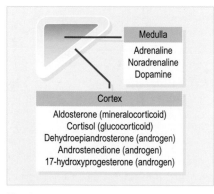

Fig. 1 **The relationship between the adrenal cortex and medulla, and their main hormones.**

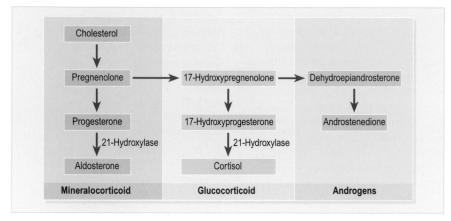

Fig. 2 **The major adrenal steroids and pathways. Note that not all precursors or pathways are shown.**

and sometimes a splenectomy is necessary. Both adrenals take arterial supplies from several branches from the aorta, renal and phrenic arteries.

Adrenal cortex

Physiology

Adrenal steroids are manufactured in a series of enzymatic steps (Fig. 2), using cholesterol as a substrate. Three main types of steroid hormone are made:

- glucocorticoids
- mineralocorticoids
- androgens.

The main stimulator of the glucocorticoid and androgen branches is ACTH. Cortisol feeds back to inhibit corticotrophin releasing hormone and ACTH secretion from the hypothalamus and pituitary (Fig. 3).

The mineralocorticoids are primarily controlled by the salt and water balance and the kidney via the renin–angiotensin system (Fig. 4). Renin is critical to the pathway controlling aldosterone and is secreted by juxtaglomerular cells in the kidney in response to low blood volume. Renin cleaves and activates angiotensinogen, thereby stimulating the angiotensin pathway. Angiotensin II is produced as a consequence and raises blood pressure by vasoconstriction and by the stimulation of the adrenal cortex to produce aldosterone. The negative feedback regulation of renin is via the blood volume expansion caused by salt-retention by aldosterone and a direct inhibition by angiotensin II.

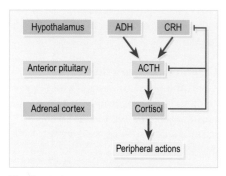

Fig. 3 **The hypothalamo–pituitary– adrenal axis and its major feedback pathway.** ADH, antidiuretic hormone; CRH, corticotrophin releasing hormone; ACTH, adrenocorticotrophic hormone.

Actions of steroid hormones

Cortisol is fat soluble and affects nearly every organ (Table 1). The pathological consequences of changes in cortisol levels (Table 2) can be predicted from its physiological effects. For example, excess cortisol over-stimulates osteoclasts and causes osteoporosis (Fig. 5).

Aldosterone acts mainly at the distal renal cortical tubule and collecting ducts to increase sodium reabsorption from the urine and decrease potassium absorption.

Aldosterone acts via an intracellular mineralocorticoid receptor. Cortisol is also able to bind the mineralocorticoid receptor. Cortisol is much more abundant than aldosterone and, based on chemical principles, should dominate the binding to the mineralocorticoid receptor. However, in aldosterone-sensitive tissues (such as the kidney), the enzyme 11 beta-hydroxysteroid

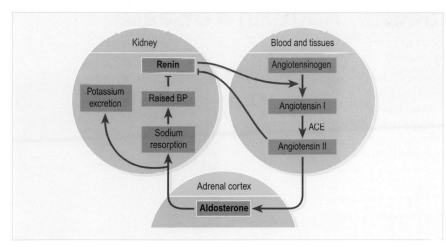

Fig. 4 The renin–angiotensin-aldosterone pathways. ACE, angiotensin converting enzyme; BP, blood pressure.

Table 1 Physiological actions of adrenal steroids

Steroid	Effect
Cortisol	Blood pressure control
	Glucose control
	Stress responses
	Lymphocyte inhibition
	Movement of neutrophils from vascular wall into bloodstream
	Thymus regression
	Osteoclast stimulation
Aldosterone	Salt retention
	Potassium excretion
	Proton (acid) excretion
Dehydroepiandrosterone/ androstenedione	Muscle maintenance
	Bone anabolism
	Mental drive
	Sexual function

Table 2 Diseases associated with defective adrenal function

Dysfunction	Disease
Cortisol excess	Cushing's syndrome; (p. 28)
Cortisol deficiency	Addison's disease (p. 24)
Aldosterone excess	Conn's syndrome (p. 26)
General steroid hormone excess	Adrenal adenomas (p. 30)
Noradrenaline and adrenaline excess	Phaeochromocytomas (p. 32)

dehydrogenase is expressed and converts cortisol to cortisone. Cortisone cannot bind the mineralocorticoid receptor, thereby allowing aldosterone to act specifically at the receptor.

Adrenal medulla

Physiology

The adrenal medulla is part of the sympathetic nervous system, which, in turn, is part of the autonomic nervous system. The medulla is essentially a

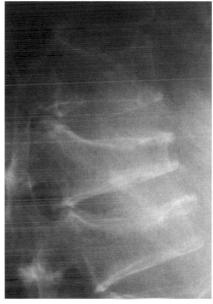

Fig. 5 Vertebral osteoporotic crush fractures at multiple levels. The patient is at risk of spinal stenosis or compression.

large ganglion, receiving preganglionic axons from the spinal cord via the greater splanchnic nerve. Activation of adrenal medullary action occurs mainly in response to stress. The postganglionic neural tissue in the medulla manufactures and secretes the catecholamines, adrenaline and

noradrenaline. Adrenaline is about twice as abundant as noradrenaline, as the medullary enzyme phenylethanolamine-N-methyltransferase converts noradrenaline to adrenaline. This conversion is unique to the adrenal medulla as the enzyme is induced by the high local cortisol concentrations diffusing from the adjacent adrenal cortex.

Actions of catecholamines

The overall action of catecholamines is the response to stress ('fight and flight'). The heart beats faster and stronger, and blood pressure and blood sugar rise. There is reduced blood flow to non-vital organs, dilatation of the pupils and airways, and increased sweating. These actions of catecholamines are mediated by adrenoreceptors, which are found on the surface of cells. The receptors have specific and different actions depending on their second messenger intracellular signalling pathways. A central negative feedback pathway is mediated by the α_2-adrenoceptor, which is situated on nerve terminals. When stimulated, these receptors inhibit nerve terminal action, with a consequent lowering of sympathetic outflow from the central nervous system. The physiological actions of catecholamines depend on the adrenoceptor involved (Table 3).

Table 3 Physiological actions of catecholamines

Receptor	Actions
α_1	Vasoconstriction
	Blood pressure maintenance
	Glucose maintenance
	Cardiac contraction and tachycardia
	Sweating, especially palms
	Piloerection 'hair standing on end'
α_2	Sympathetic outflow inhibition
	Insulin secretion inhibition
	Vasoconstriction
β_1	Cardiac contraction and tachycardia
	Renin secretion stimulation
β_2	Vasodilatation
	Smooth muscle relaxation
	Glucose maintenance

Adrenal glands and endocrine hypertension

- The adrenal cortex makes steroid hormones.
- The adrenal medulla makes catecholamines.
- Cortisol is the main glucocorticoid.
- Aldosterone is the main mineralocorticoid.
- Adrenaline is the main catecholamine.
- Androgens are also produced.
- Adrenal hormones increase plasma glucose, blood pressure and salt retention.

Primary hypoadrenalism: Addison's disease

Causes

Hypoadrenalism is classified into *primary* (failure of the adrenal itself) or *secondary* (caused by deficiency of ACTH). Primary hypoadrenalism is uncommon. The prevalence was 6:100 000 in North East Thames region of the UK. There are two common causes of primary hypoadrenalism:

- autoimmune
  - cause of 80% of cases
  - gives cortical atrophy only
  - anti-adrenal antibodies usually present
- tuberculosis
  - whole gland involved
  - calcification on radiograph or computed tomography (CT)
  - becoming more common.

The female-to-male ratio of 2:1 reflects the autoimmune aetiology. Autoimmune destruction usually affects the adrenal cortex and spares the medulla, while tuberculous adrenalitis affects both medulla and cortex. Tuberculous adrenalitis is becoming more common in the UK (Fig. 1). The likelihood of tuberculosis of the adrenal increases as the incidence of general tuberculous infections increases in the community. In communities where tuberculosis is endemic, tuberculous adrenalitis is a very common cause of primary hypoadrenalism. Similarly, histoplasmosis adrenalitis should be considered in a patient from an endemic area. As 80–90% of both adrenals must be affected to destroy adrenal reserve, other causes are rare.

Rare causes include:

- adrenal haemorrhage (usually in septicaemic patients or those taking anticoagulants and often missed)
- adrenoleukodystrophy
- amyloidosis
- congenital adrenal hyperplasia
- drugs (e.g, metirapone, mitotane, ketoconazole)
- familial glucocorticoid deficiency (caused by an ACTH receptor mutation)
- hemochromatosis
- HIV-related adrenalitis
- metastases and lymphoma
- sarcoidosis
- histoplasmosis (patient may have travelled in Ohio or Mississippi river basins or Southern USA).

Symptoms and signs

The onset is often insidious. The diagnosis may be delayed by the non-specific nature of the symptoms:

- weakness, fatigue, weight loss (very common)
- pigmentation, persistent tan after a holiday (common)
- gut symptoms (in about 50%)
- dizziness and syncope
- musculoskeletal pain, symmetrical (in < 10%)
- mental changes
- acute back pain in patient taking anticoagulants (rare).

However, hypoadrenalism is easily tested for, and completely treatable, so it is a diagnosis that should be considered often. Furthermore, acute circulatory collapse may be precipitated by any physical stress in a patient with poor or fixed adrenal function. Therefore, once considered, action should be taken to confirm or refute the diagnosis.

Signs

By the time cardiovascular signs of the disease have appeared, the hypoadrenalism is severe and there is a

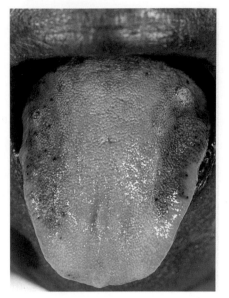

Fig. 3 **Addisonian pigmentation on the sides of the tongue and upper lip.**

risk of imminent circulatory collapse. Signs are:

- postural hypotension
- hypotension, usually systolic blood pressure is < 110 mmHg
- pigmentation, often generalized, but check extensor and exposed skin (common; Fig. 2)
- buccal pigmentation (Fig. 3), usually present with generalized pigmentation
- scar pigmentation: in primary hypoadrenalism, pigmentation is classically on areas of trauma sustained after disease onset
- signs of other organ-specific autoimmune disease (vitiligo, thyroid signs)
- signs of rare diseases such as short stature (congenital adrenal hyperplasia), neurological signs (adrenoleukodystrophy or amyloidosis), hypogonadism and liver signs (haemochromatosis).

Investigations

The simplest test is a serum cortisol (Table 1). In primary hypoadrenalism, the adrenal gland will fail to produce cortisol even after prolonged administration of synthetic ACTH (tetracosactide; Synacthen) at high doses. Conversely, in secondary forms caused by ACTH deficiency, the adrenal will recover and produce a cortisol rise after the prolonged

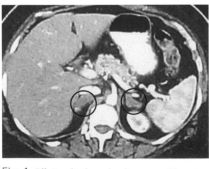

Fig. 1 **Bilateral adrenal enlargement in tuberculous adrenalitis (circled).**

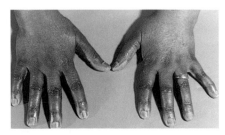

Fig. 2 **Addisonian pigmentation over extensor skin creases.**

Table 1 Abnormal tests in primary hypoadrenalism

Tests	Comment
Serum cortisol	Simplest test. Cortisol level is usually at least 500 nmol/L in a normal subject undergoing physical stress; It is < 200 nmol/L in a patient with severe hypoadrenalism (the occasional patient with partial hypoadrenalism may have 200–500 nmol/L during acute illness)
Serum sodium	Hyponatraemia: inability to excrete water caused by raised ADH (common)
Serum potassium	Hyperkalaemia: usually mild (may be normal in 40% of cases)
Serum calcium	Hypercalcaemia: in < 10%
Serum glucose	Hypoglycaemia, sometimes seen in children or undernourished patients
Blood count and film	Eosinophilia; macrocytosis with coexistent vitamin B_{12} deficiency; normocytic anaemia after volume replacement
Chest X-ray	Look for tuberculosis
Plasma ACTH	Usually > 50 ng/L (NB, centrifuge and freeze sample immediately)
Plasma renin	High
Plasma aldosterone	Low

Box 1 Synacthen tests

There are no contraindications, no precautions and Synacthen tests can be done in non-fasting patients. Note that the cortisol ranges depend on the assay used.

Short Synacthen test

Tetracosactide 250 µg intramuscular. Measure cortisol at 0, 30 and 60 minutes (normal rise > 580 nmol/L, with an increment of 200 nmol/L). This will not distinguish primary from secondary adrenal failure.

Long Synacthen test

Tetracosactide depot 1 mg intramuscular daily. Measure serum cortisol at 0, 30, 60, 90, 120 minutes and 4, 6, 8, 12, 24, 48 and 72 hours. In secondary adrenal failure, the cortisol usually starts to rise by 24 hours with a cortisol > 580 nmol/L by 72 hours. In primary adrenal failure no rise occurs. The cortisol values of the short and long Synacthen tests at 0, 30, and 60 minutes are usually very similar.

Box 2 Management of hypoadrenalism

Immediate management

Once considered, this diagnosis *must* be acted upon. If the patient is acutely sick or hypotensive:

- Take blood for cortisol, glucose, urea and electrolytes
- Give *hydrocortisone* 100 mg as intravenous bolus
- Give *saline* infusion 1 litre initially over 4–6 hours
- Correct hypoglycaemia with intravenous boluses of 20% glucose.

NB Inotropic agents will not work unless cortisol is replaced.

Continue with *hydrocortisone* 100 mg intramuscular 6 hourly (longer half life when given intramuscular) until clinically improved. Patients in intensive care or receiving anticoagulants can be treated with a hydrocortisone infusion (100 mg in 50 mL saline given at 2 mg/h).

Long-term management

Refer to specialist endocrine unit. All patients should have 24 hour direct access to such a centre.

- Hydrocortisone orally 10 mg on waking, 5 mg at lunch and evening (dose varies).
- Fludrocortisone 0.1–0.2 mg per day.
- Supply a steroid warning card, Medicalert bracelet (Fig. 4), and 'emergency pack' (hydrocortisone 100 mg ampoule with saline, 21-guage needle and 2 mL syringe).
- Teach the partner how to give an intramuscular injection in case of vomiting or coma.
- Educate the patient about the need for extra hydrocortisone in case of illness (e.g. gastroenteritis) or physical stress (surgery).

administration of Synacthen. Note that in partial ACTH deficiency, there may be a normal adrenal response even during the short Synacthen test (Box 1).

Management

Treatment is for life and is best with hydrocortisone (the pharmaceutical name for cortisol) and a synthetic derivative of aldosterone (fludrocortisone) (Box 2). The morning tablets should be taken on waking, well before breakfast. Oral hydrocortisone is fully detected by the cortisol assay and levels can be monitored at timed intervals after taking the tablets. The serum cortisol level should peak at 800–1000 nmol/L, with a level before the evening dose not lower than 100 nmol/L. Plasma renin activity should be measured 2 hours after the fludrocortisone dose and maintained in the normal range.

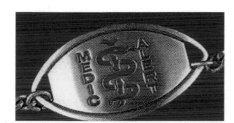

Fig. 4 **The Medicalert bracelet.**

Addison's disease

- Onset of symptoms is often insidious.
- Patients are often pigmented.
- Cortisol is usually low.
- ACTH is elevated.
- Commonest cause is autoimmune adrenalitis in western countries.
- Treatment is with hydrocortisone and fludrocortisone.

Conn's syndrome

Conn's syndrome is a disease of the adrenal glands involving excess production of aldosterone. This condition is also called *primary hyperaldosteronism*. Conn's syndrome is a potentially curable cause of hypertension. It is an underdiagnosed condition. Some studies suggest that Conn's syndrome is rare (one new case in a million population each year). However, when detailed investigations have been performed in patients with hypertension, up to 15% may have a biochemical pattern of primary hyperaldosteronism.

Pathogenesis

The excess secretion of aldosterone has two main sources: from a benign cortical adrenal adenoma (Fig. 1) or from hyperplasia of both adrenals. An adenoma is surgically curable, while hyperplasia is not. The underlying reasons for the development of an adenoma or hyperplasia are not known. Damage to genes in the adrenal gland may be an early step, as in other tumours. Some families with multiple endocrine neoplasia (MEN) type I (p. 48) have an increased likelihood of developing an adrenocortical adenoma.

The endocrinological behaviour of an aldosterone-producing adenoma is different from hyperplasia. The physiological controls of aldosterone secretion are:

- circulating blood volume, salt and water (primary control)
  — reflected in the effect of changes in posture

- adrenocorticotrophin (ACTH; secondary control)
  — reflected in a circadian rhythm.

In patients with hyperplasia, the normal aldosterone response to changing posture from lying to standing is exaggerated and the serum aldosterone nearly always rises. By contrast, in aldosterone-producing adenomas, the physiological control of circulating volume and salt and water is less. Instead, adenomas are often more responsive to ACTH. The ACTH level usually falls during the day as part of the circadian rhythm, and so does the aldosterone level during the time course of postural studies in adenomas, even if the patient is tested while standing.

Symptoms and signs

Hypertension is the main, and often the only, symptom. Other symptoms may occur because high serum aldosterone levels act at the distal renal tubule to increase the loss of potassium in the urine. This, in turn, may lead to hypokalaemia, resulting in tiredness, muscle weakness, polyuria and nocturia. Polyuria and nocturia result from renal resistance to antidiuretic hormone (ADH) (nephrogenic diabetes insipidus) induced by hypokalaemia. However, these symptoms are not specific to Conn's syndrome and are found in many other conditions (for example, diabetes mellitus or hypercalcaemia). Note that many patients with proven Conn's syndrome do not have hypokalaemia.

Investigations

A major difficulty is who to investigate, because Conn's syndrome may be suspected in all patients with high blood pressure. Traditional teaching has been to investigate only patients who have hypokalaemia, in whom blood pressure is moderate to severe (> 160/110 mmHg) or where several

drugs are needed to control hypertension. However, using these criteria, many patients with Conn's syndrome will not be diagnosed. For example, about 40% of patients with proven Conn's syndrome have normal plasma potassium levels.

Investigations include:

- plasma urea, electrolytes
- plasma bicarbonate and chloride
- serum aldosterone
- plasma renin
- urine sodium and potassium
- lying and standing aldosterone
- CT of adrenals (high resolution).

The first step is to test the electrolytes, bicarbonate and renal function as a hypokalaemic alkalosis is classically present in Conn's syndrome. The finding of a normal plasma potassium does not exclude Conn's syndrome. This may be because some patients will have reduced the intake of salt in their diet on their own initiative or on medical advice and the reduced renal salt load decreases the loss of potassium in the urine and normalizes the plasma potassium. In addition, blood samples are often haemolyzed and the potassium leak from red cells falsely elevates the potassium level. In such cases, the plasma bicarbonate may be unaffected and remains elevated.

A single blood sample to measure the ratio of aldosterone to renin has increased the number of patients treated for Conn's syndrome. In theory, the aldosterone to renin ratio (ARR) is a convenient test to screen patients presenting with hypertension. In practice, the optimal conditions of posture or sample time for measuring the ARR are unclear. Anti-hypertensive drugs, salt and liquorice intake can affect the ARR (see below). In addition, renin measurement techniques are either plasma renin activity or direct renin concentration immunoassays, and the latter may be imprecise at the lower end of the normal range. The

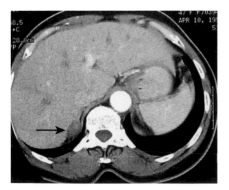

Fig. 1 **Computed tomography of the right adrenal gland showing an adrenocortical adenoma secreting aldosterone.**

Table 1 **Drugs and the renin–aldosterone system**	
Drug	**Effect**
Angiotensin-converting enzyme (ACE) inhibitors	Elevation of renin
Angiotensin II receptor blockers	Elevation of renin
Beta-adrenoceptor blockers	Suppression of renin
Diuretics	Salt depletion, hypokalaemic alkalosis, elevation of renin

ARR value will depend on the units used to express aldosterone and renin levels, and on the technique used in the hospital's laboratory.

- ARR suggestive of Conn's syndrome:
  S.I. units: aldosterone (pmol/L): renin activity (pmol/L/hr) > 800
  Conventional units: aldosterone (ng/dL): renin activity (ng/ml/h) > 67
- ARR indicating Conn's syndrome is unlikely:
  S.I. units: aldosterone (pmol/L): renin activity (pmol/L/hr) < 300
  Conventional units: aldosterone (ng/dL): renin activity (ng/ml/h) < 24

The most rigorous method of diagnosis is to measure serum aldosterone levels and plasma renin activity during postural studies. The serum aldosterone is usually elevated and the plasma renin is nearly always subnormal or undetectable. Postural studies may be simply done as follows:

- 0830 h: start with the patient lying down
- 0900-h: take blood for lying aldosterone, cortisol and renin
- 0900-h to 1200-h: allow patient to move freely
- 1200-h to 1300-h: patient remains constantly upright
- 1300-h: take blood for standing aldosterone, cortisol and renin.

The main problem with interpreting postural studies is that patients may become physically stressed by standing for long periods of time. This may result in a high ACTH drive and thus elevated aldosterone levels from an adenoma.

The interpretation of the tests requires some care, particularly in the light of medications (Table 1). For example, a hypokalaemic alkalosis may be caused by a loss of potassium in the urine as a result of diuretic treatment of essential hypertension. Renin levels may be suppressed by some drugs that are commonly used to treat hypertension (most notably β-adrenoceptor blockers) and this may lead to an incorrect diagnosis of primary hyperaldosteronism. Our practice is to convert the patient to long-acting calcium channel blockers

(such as amlodipine) for 3 weeks and prescribe a salt intake of 120 mEq/day for 3 days prior to specific tests of the renin–aldosterone axis.

The distinction between a single, unilateral aldosterone-producing adenoma and bilateral hyperplasia (or idiopathic hyperaldosteronism) is based on a combination of tests. These include lying and standing aldosterone, renin and cortisol measurements, CT or magnetic resonance imaging (MRI) of the adrenals and occasionally adrenal vein sampling for aldosterone.

Thus, a unilateral adenoma will have the following investigations:

- aldosterone falls in the postural study
- CT or MRI adrenals shows single nodule
- high aldosterone from one adrenal vein.

Rare diseases that clinically mimic Conn's syndrome can be distinguished by careful biochemical testing:

- glucocorticoid-suppressible hyperaldosteronism
- adrenal cancers (very rarely make aldosterone with other steroids)
- Liddle's disease: serum aldosterone levels low
- excessive liquorice intake: serum aldosterone levels low
- 11β-hydroxysteroid dehydrogenase type 2 mutations: serum aldosterone levels low
- abnormal deoxycorticosterone secretion: serum aldosterone levels low.

Management
Potassium supplements may be needed and some patients (with plasma potassium < 2.5 mmol/L)

warrant urgent inpatient treatment. Aldosterone receptor blockers (spironolactone) or potassium-sparing diuretics are important agents after biochemical confirmation of the diagnosis. Spironolactone is similar in chemical structure to oestradiol, and a major side-effect is painful gynaecomastia in men. Therefore, other potassium-retaining drugs (amiloride or triamterene) may be combined with a lower dose of spironolactone. Laboratory animals treated over long periods with very high doses of spironolactone have developed tumours, but this has not been a problem in humans, despite several decades of clinical experience. A selective aldosterone receptor blocker called eplerenone is now available and does not have oestrogenic side-effects.

Definitive treatment for an aldosterone-producing adenoma is surgical removal (unilateral adrenalectomy). This may be performed via laparoscopic approaches, with shorter hospital stays compared with open surgery. After adrenalectomy, many patients with a single adrenal adenoma will be able to stop drug treatment and will have normal blood pressures.

Surgery will fail to cure Conn's syndrome that is caused by bilateral hyperplasia, and long-term medical treatment is required. Aldosterone-receptor blockade is central to control of blood pressure and preservation and repair of cardiac muscle function. Spironolactone or eplerenone doses may be assessed by clinic blood pressure measurement, plasma electrolyte and renal function and 24-h ambulatory blood pressure recording.

Conn's syndrome
- Conn's syndrome is caused by primary hyperaldosteronism and presents with hypertension.
- Classically, hypokalaemic alkalosis is found.
- Plasma renin is low.
- Aldosterone-producing adenomas are cured by adrenalectomy.
- Bilateral adrenal hyperplasia is treated medically.

Cushing's syndrome

Cushing's syndrome is the clinical state caused by excess levels of corticosteroids. The commonest cause is the use of exogenous corticosteroids to treat steroid-responsive diseases. The main classification of endogenous Cushing's syndrome is into ACTH-dependent and ACTH-independent causes (Table 1). Cushing's disease is caused by a pituitary adenoma oversecreting ACTH. In Cushing's disease and other ACTH-dependent causes, generalized adrenocortical hyperplasia results in abnormal levels of adrenal androgens. By contrast, adrenal adenomas secreting cortisol only will suppress ACTH and the activity of the remaining adrenal cortex, resulting in low or undetectable adrenal androgens. The mortality of untreated Cushing's syndrome is as high as 50% in 5 years and is most commonly caused by infections and cardiovascular complications. Ectopic ACTH syndrome arises from neoplasms of non-pituitary origin, usually a small cell lung carcinoma or neuroendocrine tumours from a variety of organs.

Symptoms and signs

Cushing's syndrome has a wide range of presentations depending on the aetiology and severity.

Symptoms

The presentation of Cushing's syndrome can be with:

- weight gain resistant to dieting
- change in body and facial shape
- thin and easily bruised skin
- muscle weakness
- hirsutism and acne
- balding
- labile mood or depression
- sexual dysfunction
- menstrual irregularity
- sleep disturbance
- osteoporotic fracture/vertebral collapse
- increased infections
- poor wound healing
- kidney stones

- anorexia and weight loss
- pigmentation
- incidentally discovered pituitary/adrenal mass
- polycystic ovary syndrome
- hypertension
- type II diabetes mellitus.

The secretory activity of the adenoma or tumour may vary, causing spontaneous and temporary remissions (also called 'cyclical' Cushing's syndrome). The excess of cortisol affects every tissue. Classically there is an insidious onset. However, patients with severe ectopic ACTH syndrome may experience a rapid onset of weakness (caused by severe hypokalaemic alkalosis) and pigmentation (caused by high plasma ACTH stimulating melanocyte-stimulating hormone receptors). A significant percentage of female patients with milder Cushing's syndrome have a similar presentation to polycystic ovary syndrome (p. 40). Occasionally an alert physician will identify Cushing's

syndrome in a patient presenting with type II diabetes mellitus or hypertension, because of additional symptoms or signs. An increasingly common presentation is the finding of an adrenal or pituitary mass during scanning for another indication, leading to investigations showing Cushing's syndrome.

Signs

The classical signs are:

- central and truncal obesity (e.g. 'buffalo hump', a fat accumulation between the scapulae), with thin legs and arms caused by proximal muscle myopathy ('lemon on a stick' appearance; Fig. 1)
- livid or purple striae and easy bruising may be striking (Fig. 2)
- the face is plethoric with a rounded shape ('moon face').

Other signs are thin skin, proximal muscle weakness, hypertension, hirsutism, skin infections or poor wound healing.

Many patients do not have classical signs and studying old photographs may help (Fig. 3). Infections are common but particularly difficult to diagnose because fever and local inflammatory signs may be suppressed by high cortisol levels.

Investigations

Numerous abnormalities may be found:

- polycythaemia, neutrophilia
- hypokalaemia, alkalosis
- elevated plasma glucose
- HbA1c (glycosylated haemoglobin A1c) elevation
- hyperlipidaemia
- urine microbiology for infection
- chest X-ray for infection

Table 1 **Classification of Cushing's syndrome**	
Source of excess corticosteroids	**Cause**
Exogenous	Therapy
Endogenous	
ACTH independent	Adrenocortical adenoma, adrenocortical carcinoma, primary adrenal nodular hyperplasias (rare)
ACTH dependent	Pituitary adenoma (Cushing's disease), ectopic ACTH syndrome (rare)

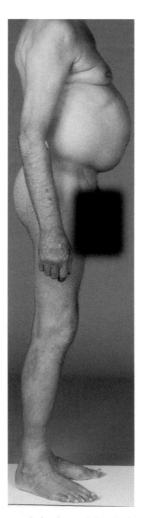

Fig. 1 **Central obesity and thin limbs.** Note the curvature of the spine caused by osteoporotic vertebral crush fractures.

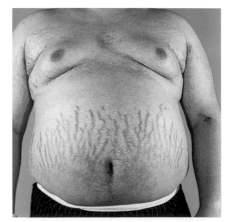

Fig. 2 **Livid broad striae, truncal obesity and bruising (left antecubital fossa).**

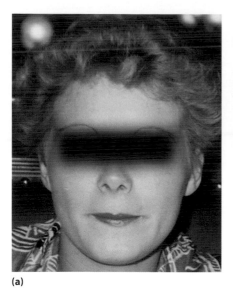 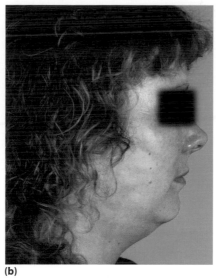 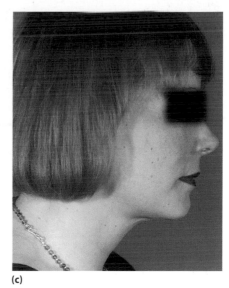

(a)   (b)   (c)

Fig. 3   **Facial shape in a patient with Cushing' disease: (a) prior to onset; (b) at the time of diagnosis; (c) after cure.**

- spine X-ray for fractures
- DEXA (dual energy X-ray absorptiometry) bone mineral density.

Multiple fractures may be notable in men (Fig. 5, p. 23). Blood, urine and sputum cultures, chest X-ray, abdominal ultrasound and CT should be available in any patient with Cushing's syndrome who becomes unwell or who has a tachycardia or hypotension, because of the dangers of a masked infection.

The next aim is to confirm an excess of circulating cortisol (Table 2). Patients should not be tested while acutely unwell with another condition (for example, cardiac failure). The physiological response to illness will give high cortisol levels, which may be misinterpreted as Cushing's syndrome. In Cushing's syndrome, serum cortisol levels are detectable (> 50 nmol/L) while asleep at midnight or after low doses of dexamethasone (Box 1). Note that while serum and urine cortisol levels are often high in classical or severe forms, they may be normal in borderline cases and there is no simple out-patient screening test that will reliably exclude Cushing's syndrome.

Box 1   The low-dose dexamethasone suppression test

1. Measure serum cortisol at 0900 h before dexamethasone on day 0.
2. Patient takes oral dexamethasone 0.5 mg at 0900 h, 1500 h, 2100 h and 0300 h for 48 hours on day 0 and day 1.
3. Measure 0900 h serum cortisol on day 2.

The main principle of locating the site of Cushing's syndrome is that an undetectable plasma ACTH suggests primary adrenal disease. A pitfall is the incorrect handling of the blood sample for ACTH, which is subject to rapid degradation. In ACTH-dependent Cushing's disease, serum cortisol levels usually change in response to dynamic tests with dexamethasone or corticotrophin-releasing hormone. This is because pituitary adenomas often retain some feedback regulation. By contrast, ectopic ACTH syndrome will usually show no response to dynamic tests. Hypokalaemic alkalosis is a feature of very high serum cortisol levels and immediately suggests ectopic ACTH syndrome.

Management

Control of infections, hypokalaemia, hyperglycaemia, hypertension and psychiatric manifestations are essential early on. Several specific medical treatments are available to block the production of cortisol:

- ketoconazole (a steroidogenic pathway blocker)
- metirapone (a 11β-hydroxylase blocker)
- mitotane (an adrenolytic drug).

Patients with severe Cushing's syndrome should be treated medically for 6 weeks prior to surgery to allow better tissue healing after surgery.

Cure is by excision of the tumour. This is by transsphenoidal hypophysectomy for Cushing's disease or adrenalectomy for a cortisol-secreting adrenal adenoma. All patients should be covered with corticosteroids for surgery as a surgical cure will render them immediately hypoadrenal. Hydrocortisone replacement will then be needed for months or years until recovery of the endogenous axis.

Other treatments include bilateral adrenalectomy or pituitary radiotherapy, where localization or removal of the primary tumour is not possible.

Table 2 **Tests in Cushing's syndrome**	
Confirming the syndrome	**Locating the site of the disease**
Low-dose dexamethasone suppression test (Box 1)	Paired ACTH and cortisol measurements
Midnight cortisol levels	
Serum cortisol daytime profile	Corticotrophin-releasing hormone test
24-hour urinary free cortisol	MRI of pituitary
Overnight dexamethasone suppression test	CT of adrenal glands
	Chest X-ray or CT scan
	Petrosal sinus venous sampling for ACTH

Cushing's syndrome

- Cushing's syndrome is ACTH dependent or independent.
- Cushing's disease is caused by an ACTH-secreting pituitary adenoma.
- Metabolic consequences are widespread.
- Mild or non-classical presentations are common.
- Circulating cortisol levels are high, but no simple screening test is reliable.
- Infections can be masked, so should be sought and treated aggressively.
- Medical treatment is often needed before surgery.
- Definitive treatment is surgical.

Adrenocortical adenomas and carcinomas

Adrenocortical tumours may be benign adenomas or malignant carcinomas. Functioning adrenal neoplasms secrete hormones; those that do not oversecrete a hormone are termed non-functioning. Adrenal masses are most commonly a coincidental finding during a scan of the body performed for an unrelated condition (Fig. 1), but all need careful evaluation to ascertain their nature and function. The cause of sporadic adrenal adenomas is not known, but they probably arise because of mutations in key genes. Adrenal adenomas are more common in some inherited diseases:

- multiple endocrine neoplasia type I
- congenital adrenal hyperplasia (poorly controlled)
- Beckwith–Wiedemann syndrome
- Carney complex.

The likelihood of discovering an adenoma increases with age; approximately 6% of patients over 60 years of age may harbour an adrenal adenoma. Benign adrenal adenomas are found in about 5% of autopsy studies.

Symptoms and signs

The majority of patients will have no symptoms attributable to the adenoma. However, even in these patients, some adrenal adenomas have subtle abnormalities of steroid hormone oversecretion when properly investigated. The commonest is an excess of cortisol; even minimal oversecretion has been associated with weight problems, hypertension and diabetes mellitus. Some adenomas will cause frank symptoms because of massive oversecretion of steroid hormones. Large excesses of cortisol will cause Cushing's syndrome (p. 28); excesses of aldosterone cause Conn's syndrome (p. 26), and excesses of male sex steroids cause acne and hair growth.

Very rarely, bleeding may occur into adenomas and cause pain in the flanks or back.

Investigations

Most are incidentally discovered when an abdominal CT or MRI scan is performed because of unrelated symptoms. CT scanning identifies an incidental adrenal mass in 0.3–11% of patients. About 80% will be benign non-functioning adrenocortical adenomas. Carcinomas are >6 cm and often heterogeneous in appearance (Fig. 2). Lesions secreting androgens are more likely to be carcinomas. Carcinomas metastasize to lungs, liver and bones often via the adrenal vein and inferior vena cava. Local invasion may be present.

A mass in the adrenal could be a metastasis from a cancer in another organ (usually the lung or bowel). Generally the origin of the cancer is clear from the history, clinical examination or simple tests such as a chest radiograph. The CT or MR appearance of metastatic cancer in the adrenal can be distinguished from a benign adrenal adenoma. Adrenal masses may also be phaeochromocytomas (p. 32)

Imaging cannot distinguish between functioning and non-functioning adrenal lesions and endocrine testing is essential:

- urea, electrolytes, plasma potassium
- lying plasma renin and aldosterone

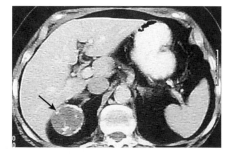

Fig. 2 **Right adrenocortical carcinoma with a large heterogeneous nature (arrow).**

- testosterone
- 17-hydroxyprogesterone
- dehydroepiandrosterone
- androstenedione
- oestradiol
- progesterone
- serum cortisol (low dose dexamethasone suppression test)
- free catecholamines: 24-hour urine collection.

Patients taking the oral contraceptive pill may be advised to stop 6 weeks before any blood tests and use barrier methods (condoms with spermicidal creams) because the oral contraceptive pill makes interpretation of circulating steroid hormones impossible.

Treatment

Adrenal lesions that are not oversecreting hormones and that have all the characteristics of a benign cortical adenoma (including size <4 cm) may be watched by scanning to ensure nothing is changing. All functioning adrenocortical adenomas should be considered for surgical treatment since this is usually curative. All patients with an excess of cortisol secretion need perioperative corticosteroid cover (see p. 25). We vaccinate patients before a left adrenalectomy, as splenectomy is a recognized complication.

Adrenal masses with uncertain characteristics on CT or MR scanning (size >4 cm, evidence of bleeding or degeneration, or a heterogeneous appearance), should be considered for removal, as they may be carcinomas. In adrenocortical carcinomas, low-dose mitotane (an adrenolytic drug) may help with symptoms and improve survival, but tumours are often refractory to chemotherapy and radiotherapy. Patients with functioning adrenocortical carcinomas gain considerable symptomatic relief if hormonal control is achieved.

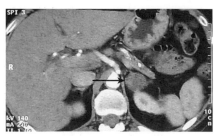

Fig. 1 **A benign non-functioning left adrenocortical adenoma (arrow) incidentally found in a patient with chronic pancreatitis.**

> *Adrenocortical adenomas and carcinomas*
>
> - Incidental adrenal masses are found in up to 10% of scans.
> - Most are adrenocortical adenomas.
> - Functioning lesions cannot be radiologically distinguished from non-functioning ones.
> - Benign and malignant lesions can usually be identified radiologically.

Congenital adrenal hyperplasia

Congenital adrenal hyperplasia (CAH) is one of the commonest genetic diseases and results from a defective enzyme in the cortisol production pathway (see Fig. 2, p. 22). The gene for 21-hydroxylase is mutated in 90% of cases. The transmission is autosomal recessive: both alleles of the gene must be abnormal. The block in cortisol production results in an accumulation of adrenal steroid precursors such as 17-hydroxyprogesterone. Circulating ACTH rises through the hypothalamo–pituitary axis response to the lowered serum cortisol level. The effect of ACTH is to drive production of steroid precursors prior to the enzyme defect and induce growth (hyperplasia) of the adrenal cortices (Fig. 1). The precursors spill over to make adrenal androgens such as dehydroepiandrosterone (DHEA) and androstenedione.

Symptoms and signs

There are three types of presentation:

- classical salt-wasting form
- classical simple virilizing form
- non-classical late onset.

The classical salt-wasting form is life threatening because of circulatory collapse and hypoglycaemia, caused by cortisol and aldosterone deficiency. The classical simple virilizing form occurs in female fetuses, with masculinization (Fig. 2) caused by the accumulation of androgenic precursors. At birth, ambiguous external genitalia are evident. The clitoris is enlarged, there is fusion of the labia, pubic hair is present (all under the influence of high androgens)

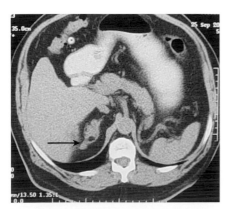

Fig. 1 **Computed tomography of adrenal glands showing hyperplasia in a poorly compliant patient. The black signal in the adrenal is an adrenomyelolipoma, a characteristic fatty mass in CAH.**

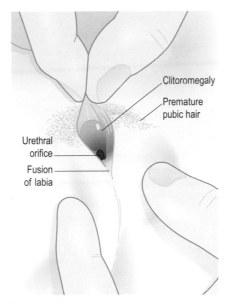

Fig. 2 **Clinical figure of a female infant patient with congenital adrenal hyperplasia.**

Clitoromegaly

Premature pubic hair

Urethral orifice

Fusion of labia

and the testes are not present (since the patients have female gonads). Virilization of females continues after birth with an early puberty and short stature. The severity of virilization does not predict the severity of salt wasting.

Androgen excess in males may become apparent later in childhood, with early puberty, short stature from premature fusion of growth plates, good skeletal muscle and penis development ('infant Hercules'). Although the penis is well developed, the testes are small and abnormal because of the production of androgens from the adrenal, which suppress the pituitary–gonadal axis. Males are vulnerable to salt wasting and circulatory collapse because the diagnosis may be missed as a result of the lack of ambiguous genitalia.

The non-classical presentation is caused by minor genetic defects with partial enzyme function and is seen in females. Symptoms begin after puberty and clinical features are often identical to polycystic ovary syndrome (hirsutism, irregular menses and acne).

Investigations

In classical salt wasting presentations, the serum sodium is low, potassium high, with an acidosis. There may be hypoglycaemia. There is a loss of salt in the urine. Serum cortisol and aldosterone are inappropriately low and plasma renin high. The diagnostic test in all classical forms is elevated serum

17-hydroxyprogesterone. In non-classical forms, the unstimulated serum 17-hydroxyprogesterone may be normal, however, there will be an exaggerated rise after stimulation with Synacthen (synthetic ACTH) Box 1, p. 25.

Genetic testing is useful is assessing the risks of having a baby with CAH. As a patient with CAH will transmit one allele to the fetus, the fetus will at least be a carrier of a mutated allele. The child will only have CAH if the other parent is a carrier of a mutated allele and if this allele is inherited by the fetus. The risks are much greater in consanguineous parents. Even where parents are unrelated, carriers of mutations in the 21-hydroxylase gene may be found commonly in some populations. The serum 17-hydroxyprogesterone level in the cord blood is measured at birth to confirm the diagnosis.

Treatment

Treatment is with corticosteroids and mineralocorticoids in severe disease. Children are treated with small doses, and serum 17-hydroxyprogesterone, growth and development are monitored. In pregnancies with a high risk of CAH, fetal adrenal hyperplasia and virilization of the external genitalia can be prevented by treating the mother with the synthetic corticosteroid dexamethasone, which crosses the placenta. In non-classical disease, small doses of night-time steroids may suppress the high ACTH, reduce adrenocortical hyperplasia and improve symptoms. One regimen in adults is to use plain prednisolone 5 mg last thing at night to suppress ACTH and then 2.5 mg on waking to prevent hypoadrenalism.

Congenital adrenal hyperplasia

- CAH is an autosomal recessive disease.
- Presents at birth through to young adult age.
- CAH causes virilization in females.
- There is a wide range of severity
- Serum 17-hydroxyprogesterone accumulates.
- CAH is treated with adrenal steroid replacement.

Phaeochromocytoma and paraganglioma

Phaeochromocytomas are neoplasms of the adrenal medulla and originate from chromaffin cells. Chromaffin cells are named after the chemical (chromate) that stains them a brown colour on histological slides. Most phaeochromocytomas secrete excessive noradrenaline (norepinephrine) and adrenaline (epinephrine). However, some secrete ectopic peptide hormones, and some do not produce any hormones. Paragangliomas are similar tumours histologically and are also of chromaffin cell origin. Paragangliomas may be situated along the entire sympathetic chain, from the base of the skull to the bottom of the pelvis. Paragangliomas commonly occur in the second to third decades in both men and women and are less often hormonally active than pheochromocytomas. They secrete noradrenaline and rarely dopamine. The commonest sites of paragangliomas are the para-aortic region at the level of the renal hila (46%), at the organ of Zukerkandl (29%), in the thoracic paraspinal region (10%), the bladder (10%) and the head and neck (2–4%). In the head and neck, 80% are carotid body or glomus vagal tumours. Paragangliomas are more likely to be malignant (40%) than phaeochromocytomas (2–11%). The classical rule of 10s is useful to remember for phaeochromocytomas:

- 10% are malignant
- 10% are extra-adrenal (paragangliomas)
- 10% are bilateral
- 10% are familial.

However, recent studies suggest familial disease occurs in up to 30% of patients presenting with phaeochromocytomas and paragangliomas (Table 1).

Symptoms and signs

Many patients with phaeochromocytomas die of the condition and the diagnosis is made at autopsy. The cardinal feature is *hypertension* (Fig. 1). This is often labile and need not be sustained. So a normal blood pressure does not exclude the diagnosis. There is often an additional clinical feature, such as:

- sweating
- palpitations
- faintness
- altered bowel habit
- weight loss, fever.
- headaches
- anxiety
- abdominal pain

A tachycardia during a blood pressure surge should raise suspicion. An

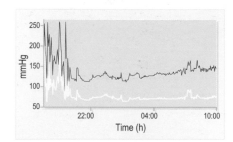

Fig. 1 **Blood pressure trace showing hypertensive surges in a patient with a phaeochromocytoma until treatment control at 2100 hours (red-systolic; white-diastolic).**

increasingly common presentation is as an incidental finding of an adrenal mass during abdominal scanning. Presentation with a crisis of extreme hypertension, paralytic ileus and cardiac failure may be triggered by manipulation or biopsy of the tumour or other physical stresses. Features of underlying genetic diseases may be present (Table 1).

Phaeochromocytomas may present in pregnancy. This causes significant diagnostic problems because the features are similar to pre-eclampsia. However, eclampsia is rare before the third trimester and a phaeochromocytoma should be excluded in any hypertensive pregnant patient presenting in the first or second trimester.

Investigations

All patients with labile or sustained hypertension and any of the clinical features listed above should be tested for a phaeochromocytoma. In addition to the symptoms, other features that should trigger investigation in a hypertensive patient include hyperglycaemia and low plasma potassium. There may also be an acidosis.

The commonest test is a 24-hour urine collection for free catecholamines, noradrenaline and adrenaline, or their metabolites. Measuring plasma noradrenaline and adrenaline is useful during a hypertensive crisis. A normal level of these catecholamines in a hypertensive patient makes the diagnosis very unlikely. Noradrenaline and adrenaline have short lifespans in the circulation (half life 30–120 seconds) and may also be metabolized within a tumour. Good results in diagnosing a phaeochromocytoma have been obtained by measuring plasma normetanephrine, which is a noradrenaline metabolite. If biochemical tests fail to confirm a phaeochromocytoma and yet the symptoms are suggestive, then repeat biochemical testing or CT scanning is advised.

CT or MRI scanning is very important in localizing the tumour (Fig. 4). Isotope imaging with [123I]-metaiodobenzylguanidine (MIBG) confirms the nature of the lesion. Such imaging may also identify multifocal or extra-adrenal disease (Fig. 5). A biopsy of a mass suspected of being a phaeochromocytoma or paraganglioma is rarely, if ever, needed. Bilateral or

Table 1 **Features of familial phaeochromocytomas**	
Genetic disease	**Additional features**
Multiple endocrine neoplasia type II	Medullary thyroid cancer, primary hyperparathyroidism
Von Hippel–Lindau disease	Retinal angiomas (Fig. 2), CNS haemangioblastomas, renal cell carcinomas/cysts, pancreatic cysts
Neurofibromatosis type I	Café-au-lait lesions (Fig. 3), skin neuromas, axillary freckles
Familial paraganglioma syndrome	Carotid body tumours, multiple paragangliomas Succinate dehydrogenase mutations

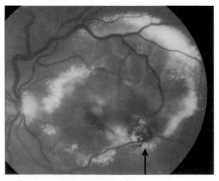

Fig. 2 **A retinal angioma (arrow) undergoing laser therapy in a patient with von Hippel–Lindau disease.**

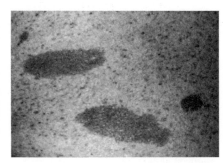

Fig. 3 **Café-au-lait lesions in neurofibromatosis type I.** The edges are smooth, in contrast to those in McCune–Albright syndrome where lesions have jagged edges.

multifocal tumours often indicate an underlying familial disease. Another sign of familial disease is young age of presentation (< 50 years of age). Care should be taken to investigate young patients, or those with a relevant family history, for other familial tumours, as these may need urgent management (Fig. 6). Genetic testing is also valuable in familial phaeochromocytoma and paraganglioma syndromes, as this allows rapid screening of relatives and an early diagnosis and presymptomatic treatment.

Elevated catecholamines may occur in other conditions, including heart failure or severe sleep apnoea. The latter may be clinically occult. Drugs that block the uptake channel, (Fig. 7) such as cocaine or certain antidepressants (desipramine), may present with a pattern identical to a phaeochromocytoma.

Management

High levels of noradrenaline are secreted from the tumour and act on adrenoceptors on postsynaptic neurons (Fig. 7). Blockade of α-adrenoceptors must be started first. The most commonly used drug is

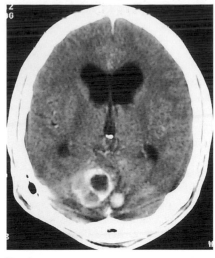

Fig. 6 **Computed tomographic head scan showing posterior fossa haemangioblastoma causing hydrocephalus in a patient with a paraganglioma and von Hippel–Lindau disease.**

phenoxybenzamine. Beta-adrenoceptor blockade is also required to protect the heart but should never be started before α-adrenoceptor blockade. Some β-adrenergic effects are vasodilatory and protect the patient from hypertension caused by α adrenergic actions. If β adrenoceptor blockers are introduced before α-adrenoceptor blockers, then unopposed α-adrenergic actions cause a worsening of hypertension.

Invasive procedures and surgery should be performed only after full adrenoreceptor blockade. Intravenous phenoxybenzamine 0.5 mg/kg in 250 ml saline is given over 2 hours every day for 72 hours prior to surgery. Treatment results in vasodilatation, haemodilution and a fall in haemoglobin. Blood transfusion to restore blood volume and haemoglobin may be needed in some patients. Experienced anaesthetic management is essential as hypertension may occur during tumour handling, followed by sudden hypotension after tumour removal. This will usually respond to volume replacement or transfusion.

Malignant lesions may be successfully treated with MIBG labelled with high radioactivity. Metastatic lesions may be very indolent and have been successfully treated with long-term α- and β-adrenoceptor blockade.

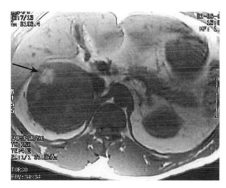

Fig. 4 **Magnetic resonance image of a right adrenal phaeochromocytoma (arrow).**

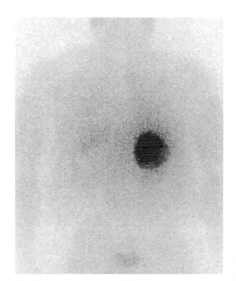

Fig. 5 **Scanning using [¹²³I]-metaiodobenzylguanidine shows uptake in right adrenal phaeochromocytoma.** View from posterior.

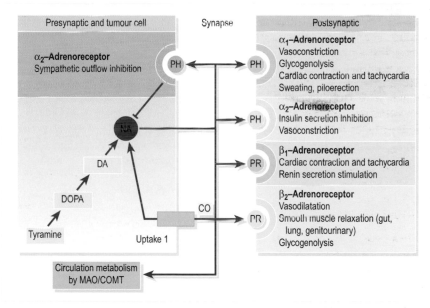

Fig. 7 **Pharmacology and metabolism of catecholamines.** Phenoxybenzamine (PH) blocks all α-adrenoreceptors; propranolol (PR) blocks all β-adrenoreceptors; cocaine (CO) blocks the uptake1 channel that takes noradrenaline (NA) from the synapse. Catecholamines spilling from the synapse are metabolized by monoamine oxidase (MAO) and catechol-O methyltransferase (COMT) in the circulation. NA is stored in secretory granules (red circle) and is made from dopamine (DA).

Phaeochromocytoma and paraganglioma

■ Phaeochromocytomas are neoplasms of the adrenal medulla; paraganglioma affect any part of the sympathetic chain.

■ Should be considered in labile hypertension.

■ Other clinical features are often present.

■ Secretory tumours may be outside the adrenal glands.

■ Therapy always starts with α-adrenergic blockers before β-blockers

■ Always use adrenergic blockade before commencing surgery to cure the patient.

Sex and fertility: basic concepts

The hypothalamus is the major control centre of the gonadal axis. Hypothalamic neurones secrete the peptide hormone gonadotrophin-releasing hormone (GnRH) into the portal circulation where it is transported to the anterior pituitary. GnRH stimulates the release of the gonadotrophins luteinizing hormone (LH) and follicle-stimulating hormone (FSH) from gonadotrophin cells in the anterior pituitary. GnRH is released in a pulsatile fashion. If GnRH is given continuously, LH and FSH are suppressed after an initial rise. This property is exploited in the therapy of hormone-sensitive tumours such as prostatic carcinoma.

LH and FSH circulate to stimulate the gonads. LH stimulates cells that make sex steroids, while FSH regulates the maturation of germ cells into ova or sperm. Gonadal sex steroids and peptide hormones exercise feedback control of the hypothalamus and pituitary (Fig. 1). In females, the sex steroids are oestradiol, progesterone, androstenedione and testosterone. In females, oestradiol has an inhibitory effect at low doses, but at high levels exerts a positive feedback on LH secretion. Testosterone is the main sex steroid in males and it exerts a negative feedback on the hypothalamus and pituitary (Fig. 2). Peptide gonadal hormones include inhibins and activins, which inhibit or activate FSH production. Multiple higher cerebral and chemical factors influence hypothalamic function and control GnRH release. Major non-hormonal inhibitors include exercise, starvation and physical and psychological stress.

Sexual differentiation

The default or constitutive state for a fetus is to develop into a female. Specific factors are required to change this and to induce male sexual differentiation (Fig. 3). The first requirement is a gene on the Y chromosome, producing testicular-determining factor, to regulate the development of undifferentiated gonads into testes. This occurs from the 7th week of fetal age onwards. Without a Y chromosome, the gonad becomes an ovary. The testes then produce testosterone under the stimulation of human chorionic gonadotrophin (HCG) from the placenta. Testosterone and dihydrotestosterone stimulate male sexual organ development between the 10th and 20th week of gestation. Müllerian-inhibiting factor is secreted by the testes to cause regression of the Müllerian structures. Defects in either testosterone or Müllerian-inhibiting factor lead to persistence of female morphology. During the second half of fetal life, the testes descend to the inguinal ring and the penis grows under the influence of dihydrotestosterone, a testosterone metabolite. The fetal hypothalamo–pituitary–gonadal axis is capable of function from the 20th week of gestation; however, full function begins at puberty.

An important but rare example of pathological development is complete androgen insensitivity syndrome (previously called testicular feminization). The androgen receptor is not functional because of mutations in the gene; there is no pubic or body hair and the external genitalia are female (Fig. 4). The gonads still function as testes, producing Müllerian inhibiting factor. The uterus and cervix are absent because of the effect of Müllerian inhibiting factor. The patient presentation is often with primary amenorrhoea. Good breast development occurs because oestrogen actions are not opposed by testosterone actions. Such complex development leads to problems in defining gender (Table 1).

Puberty

Pulsatile GnRH secretion begins at puberty, possibly triggered by a critical body size. LH and FSH levels rise and stimulate gonadal maturation plus the many changes of puberty (Table 2).

In boys, LH stimulates testosterone production from the Leydig cells and FSH stimulates the seminiferous tubules and spermatogenesis. The testes volume increases, with 90% made up of seminiferous tubules (Fig. 5). Testosterone and its metabolite

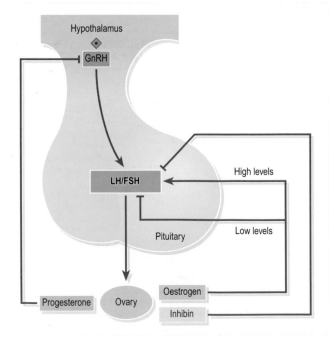

Fig. 1 **Female hypothalamo–pituitary–gonadal axis.** GnRH, gonadotrophin-releasing hormone; LH, luteinizing hormone; FSH, follicle-stimulating hormone.

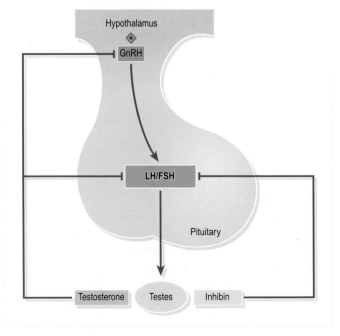

Fig. 2 **Male hypothalamo–pituitary–gonadal axis.** GnRH, gonadotrophin-releasing hormone; LH, luteinizing hormone; FSH, follicle-stimulating hormone.

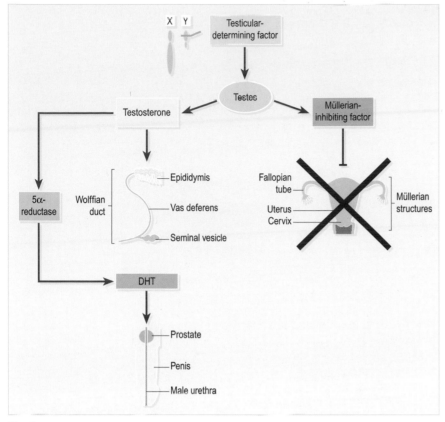

Fig. 3 **Male sexual differentiation.** The cross indicates destruction of the Müllerian structures under the influence of Müllerian-inhibiting factor.

Table 1 **Definitions of gender**	
Basis	**Feature**
Legal	Birth certificate
Chromosome content	46XX or 46XY
Gonad presence	Male with testes
	Female with ovaries
	Male pseudohermaphroditism: testes present but female sex characteristics
	Female pseudohermaphroditism: ovaries present but male sex characteristics
	True hermaphroditism: mixed gonads (ovotestes)
Phenotypic presentation	Secondary sexual characteristics
	Wolffian/Müllerian development; assessable clinically via presence of cervix

Table 2 **Terms used to describe pubertal changes**	
Term	**Definition**
Adrenarche	Pubic and axillary hair development
Gonadarche	Gonadal maturation (may be 2 years after adrenarche)
Menarche	Onset of menstrual bleeding
Thelarche	Onset of breast development
Precocious puberty (male)	Secondary sex characteristics before 9 years of age
Precocious puberty (female)	Secondary sex characteristics before 8 years
Delayed puberty (male)	No secondary sex characteristics by 15 years
Delayed puberty (female)	No secondary sex characteristics by 14 years

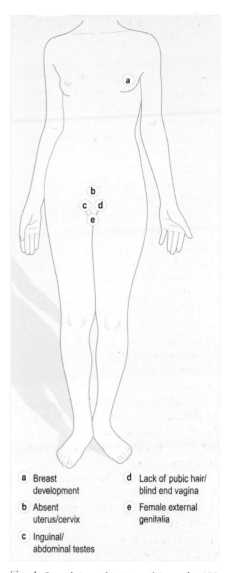

a	Breast development	d	Lack of pubic hair/ blind end vagina
b	Absent uterus/cervix	e	Female external genitalia
c	Inguinal/ abdominal testes		

Fig. 4 **Complete androgen resistance in a 46 XY patient .**

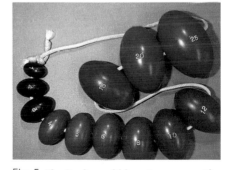

Fig. 5 **The Prader orchidometer assesses the increase in volume of the testes from prepubertal 1-3 mL to adult 15-25 mL.** The testicular tissue alone is measured by holding the epididymis away and stretching scrotal skin over the testis.

dihydrotestosterone produce male secondary sexual characteristics. The scrotal skin becomes darker and thicker, the penis grows and axillary and pubic hair develops.

In girls, LH and FSH act to stimulate oestradiol and progesterone from the theca granulosa cells. These produce breast development, fat deposition on the hips and increases in vaginal and uterine size and secretions. Pubic and axillary hair development in girls is an effect of adrenal androgens, which may occur discordantly with ovarian development. In both sexes, stimulation of the growth plates of the bones by sex steroids leads to a growth spurt that stops when the plates fuse.

Sex and fertility

- Pulsatile release of GnRH from the hypothalamus stimulates LH/FSH.
- LH stimulates sex steroid production.
- FSH stimulates germ cell maturation to sperm or ova.
- Testicular development requires testicular-determining factor on the Y chromosome.
- Ovarian development is the constitutive state.
- Testosterone and dihydrotestosterone produce male secondary sexual characteristics.

Male hypogonadism

Basic concepts

The seminiferous tubules make up 90% of the testes volumes and are devoted to spermatogenesis. Sperm develop from germ cells in the tubules supported by the Sertoli cells. Leydig cells lie close to blood vessels, between the seminiferous tubules, and produce testosterone and other sex steroids.

Local production of testosterone by Leydig cells is also important to the function of the Sertoli cell.

Testosterone action

Testosterone circulates in the blood bound to sex hormone-binding globulin (SHBG) and other proteins. About 2% of circulating testosterone is free and available for passage into cells. There is intracellular conversion of testosterone into a highly active metabolite, dihydrotestosterone, by the enzyme 5α-reductase (Fig. 1). Dihydrotestosterone binds the androgen receptor about five-times more avidly than testosterone and so there are potent dihydrotestosterone effects in tissues that express 5α-reductase, such as testis, prostate, skin, liver and kidney. Testosterone acts at every tissue.

Aetiology

The causes of hypogonadism are classified into hypogonadotrophic hypogonadism and primary hypogonadism (Table 1).

Ageing, vascular disease, diabetes mellitus, excessive exercise, obesity, physical illness, severe mental stress and drugs such as glucocorticoids are associated with hypogonadism and are common. Several genetic diseases cause hypogonadotrophic hypogonadism and are often associated with an early onset of symptoms, or the presence of associated clinical features.

Cryptorchidism is failure of the testes to descend to the bottom of the scrotum. Cryptorchidism may be idiopathic or may be associated with congenital hypogonadotrophic hypogonadism or genetic diseases (e.g. Noonan syndrome (cardiac defects and facial abnormalities)). Mumps orchitis has decreased as a result of vaccination. However, increasingly patients are seen with infections associated with the human immunodeficiency virus (HIV).

Symptoms and signs

The presenting symptoms depend on the age of onset (Table 2). Adult-onset disease is often insidious. Flushing is more frequent in patients with a more acute onset.

Signs in long-standing hypogonadism are thin, pale and finely wrinkled skin,

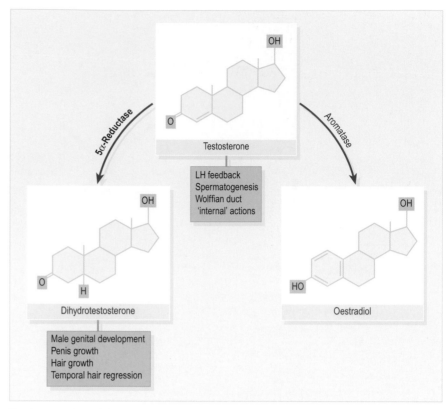

Fig. 1 **Formation of dihydrotestosterone from testosterone.**

Table 1 **Causes of hypogonadotrophic hypogonadism and primary hypogonadism**	
Hypogonadotrophic hypogonadism (hypothalamic/pituitary pathology)	**Primary hypogonadism (testicular pathology)**
Systemic diseases/stresses	Systemic diseases/stress
Pituitary or hypothalamic mass (p. 16–17)	Infections
Raised intracranial pressure	Trauma/torsion
Idiopathic isolated	Chemotherapy/radiotherapy
Haemochromatosis	Cryptorchidism
Kallmann syndrome (no smell, mirror movements, renal agenesis, midline anomalies)	Klinefelter syndrome
Prader–Willi (obesity, short stature, mental impairment)	Autoimmune
Bardet–Biedl (polydactyly, retinitis pigmentosa)	Myotonic dystrophy

and gynaecomastia. There may be evidence of osteoporotic fractures (Fig. 2). Small testes and abnormal penis anatomy are signs indicating genetic or congenital causes. Delayed fusion of the growth plate results in long arms and legs (a eunuchoid appearance) in patients with prepubertal onset of hypogonadism.

Investigation

Clinical assessment of male gonadal function includes:

- frequency of nocturnal erections
- frequency of sexual function
- frequency of spontaneous sexual thoughts
- skin thickness
- muscle strength
- gynaecomastia
- penis and urethral anatomy
- testes size
- span, height and weight.

Treatment

Testosterone replacement is safe and effective in healthy hypogonadal men.

Caution is required in patients with pre-existing diseases (Table 3). An elevated prostate-specific antigen (PSA) in a hypogonadal man is suspicious and testosterone replacement should not be started (if at all) until comprehensive assessment of the prostate.

Several routes for testosterone replacement are available, each with disadvantages (Table 4). Transdermal gels are usually well tolerated. Another approach is to start with intramuscular injections for 3 to 6 months before converting to an implant if no problems are encountered.

Table 2 **Symptoms of hypogonadism**	
Age group	**Symptoms**
Fetal/neonatal	Ambiguous genitalia, microphallus
Childhood	Delayed puberty
Adult	Sexual dysfunction, infertility, osteoporotic fractures, anaemia, flushing, fatigue

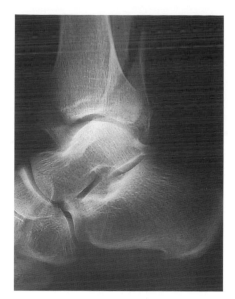

Fig. 2 **A trimalleolar osteoporotic fracture in an elderly patient presenting with Klinefelter syndrome.**

Gynaecomastia

Gynaecomastia is the presence of clinically detectable breast tissue in males (Fig. 3). Physiological gynaecomastia is very common at puberty and usually improves after a year. The development of gynaecomastia is a reflection of the balance between testosterone and oestrogens. The commonest cause of pathological gynaecomastia is drugs (Table 5).

The main clinical problem is to separate true breast tissue from fat deposition (pseudogynaecomastia). True breast tissue is attached to the nipple. When breast tissue is compressed by the examiner, the nipple will dip into the skin. The underlying cause is usually clinically evident, and simple tests will confirm these:

- exclude fatty gynaecomastia
- chest X-ray
- serum HCG and oestradiol
- serum testosterone and prolactin
- serum LH/FSH
- serum androstenedione
- serum dehydroepiandrosterone (DHEA)
- thyroxine and thyroid-stimulating hormone
- liver function tests.

Management

Surgical resection of breast tissue is required. Treatment with oestrogen receptor blockers (e.g. tamoxifen) or aromatase inhibitors (e.g. anastrozole) may be disappointing.

Klinefelter syndrome

Klinefelter syndrome is a common chromosomal abnormality with an incidence of 1:500 births. There is a

Table 3 Actions of testosterone replacement

Improved	Worsened
Libido	Polycythaemia
Sexual function	Prostatic hypertrophy
Mood	Prostatic cancer
Assertiveness	Sleep apnoea
Bone density	Aggression
Muscle mass	Truncal acne
Cholesterol	Hair loss
Anaemia	

duplication of the X chromosome (47XXY). The condition is easily missed before puberty as there are small but normal feeling prepubertal testes. At puberty there is primary hypogonadism. The presentations are with infertility and gynaecomastia. The testes are small (usually < 2 mL and always < 12 mL) and firm. The patient is eunuchoid. There is a mild testosterone deficiency in 50%, but the testosterone levels can be normal. The LH and FSH are high.

Other rare syndromes

Deficiency of 5α-reductase causes a block in the conversion of testosterone to dihydrotestosterone. The presentation is with ambiguous (female-like) genitalia at birth owing to a lack of dihydrotestosterone. There are inguinal testes, a split scrotum, a clitoral phallus and a vaginal pouch. At puberty, higher testosterone levels may result in some secondary sexual development, with scrotal testes,

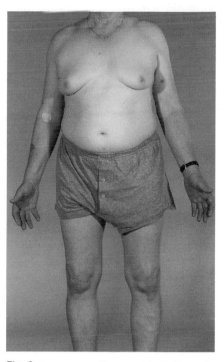

Fig. 3 **Gynaecomastia caused by Reifenstein syndrome.** Note absence of body hair, pale, bruised skin and thin thighs.

phallus growth and masculinization. The testosterone and LH are normal and there is no gynaecomastia.

Incomplete androgen resistance (**Reifenstein syndrome**) is caused by impaired testosterone receptor signalling. There is a broad spectrum of presentations including poor virilization, gynaecomastia, hypospadias, cryptorchidism, absent vas deferens and lack of sperm.

Table 4 Types of testosterone replacement

Method	Advantages	Disadvantages
Implants	Steady testosterone levels, last for 6 months	Involves a surgical procedure, pellet extrusion a risk
Intramuscular injections	Monthly dosing	Painful, peaks and troughs in testosterone levels
Transdermal	Steady testosterone levels	Allergic reactions to patches, patches may fall off, gels require daily application
Oral	Simplest to initiate	Multiple daily doses, possibility of weaker bone effects, gastrointestinal side-effects, monitoring levels difficult

Table 5 Causes of gynaecomastia

Cause	Condition
Low testosterone	Any cause of hypogonadism
High oestrogens	Testicular tumours; tumours producing increased chorionic gonadotrophin to stimulate normal testes
Increased conversion of androgens to oestrogens (by aromatase activity)	Thyrotoxicosis; obesity; increased androstenedione (aromatase substrate) in liver disease; starvation; adrenal disease
Prescribed drugs	Digoxin, spironolactone
Recreational drugs	Cannabis

Male Hypogonadism

- Hypogonadism is hypogonadotrophic or primary.
- Childhood/neonatal onset suggests a genetic cause.
- Adult-onset hypogonadism is often insidious.
- Testosterone replacement is highly effective.
- Physiological testosterone replacement may exacerbate pre-existing diseases.
- Gynaecomastia is a sign of testosterone and oestrogen imbalance or drugs.

Female hypogonadism

Female menstrual cycle

The menstrual cycle is based on the life cycle of the ovarian follicle (Fig. 1). The follicle is the principle unit of the ovary. The fetal ovary contains millions of follicles. About 400 000 follicles survive through to menarche. During the reproductive span of a female, only about 400 follicles will develop to produce ova. The follicles develop from the resting state (a primordial follicle) until a single dominant follicle is ready for ovulation on about day 14 of the cycle. This is termed the follicular phase of the cycle. After ovulation, the remaining follicle becomes the corpus luteum. The corpus luteum continues to produce high levels of progesterone for about 14 days. This is termed the luteal phase of the cycle.

Initial development of the follicle is dependent on FSH, which stimulates the production of sex steroids (oestradiol and androstenedione) from the granulosa cells. LH also stimulates sex steroid production from theca cells. The oestradiol released from the ovary increases during the follicular phase and reaches a peak in the mid cycle. The high oestradiol levels have a positive feedback on the pituitary, resulting in a sudden peak in LH secretion. The LH peak triggers breakdown of the dominant follicle, release of the ovum and formation of the corpus luteum.

Basic concepts

Between 20 and 40 years of age, the hallmark of normal ovarian function is regular uterine bleeding (Box 1). There is a wider variation in the cycle length outside this age range, although the median cycle length is unchanged. The menstrual cycle occurs in response to oestradiol and progesterone. Even minimal menstrual bleeding indicates some oestradiol activity. The uterine endometrium is primed by oestradiol in the follicular phase and bleeding occurs in response to falls in oestradiol and progesterone at the end of the luteal phase. The ovary cannot function as an endocrine gland without oocytes. Sex steroid production is from granulosa and theca cells, which are intimately related to the oocyte in the ovarian follicle. This is in contrast to the testis, where Leydig cells can produce testosterone in the absence of spermatogenesis.

Aetiology

The causes of amenorrhoea can be separated into four main classes (Table 1). Every patient should be first assumed to be pregnant, and a pregnancy test is essential. The commonest cause of hypogonadotrophic hypogonadism is weight loss. This may occur together with stress and exercise. The hypothalamo–pituitary axis is vulnerable to quite small amounts of exercise in females, with as little as 100 minutes per week having detectable effects on LH secretion in some

individuals. In such patients, there is a functional defect of the hypothalmo-pituitary–gonadal axis since resolution occurs once weight is gained and exercise reduced. A microadenoma secreting prolactin is the commonest structural hypothalamo–pituitary cause (p. 18). Polycystic ovary syndrome is not strictly associated with hypogonadism because oestradiol levels are usually normal or high (p. 40–41). However, it is a very common differential diagnosis.

Amenorrhoea can also be classified into primary or secondary: there has never been menstruation in primary amenorrhoea, whereas there has been prior menstruation in secondary amenorrhoea.

Clinical approach

A menstrual and sexual history may suggest a pregnancy. Symptoms of menopause (see below) should be sought. Weight loss, poor food intake, exercise and physical and psychological stresses may indicate a functional hypothalamo–pituitary failure. Pituitary or hypothalamic diseases may present with additional symptoms, for example galactorrhoea in patients with a prolactinoma. A drug history may reveal use of dopamine antagonists (e.g. metoclopramide in some migraine remedies), which elevate prolactin. Other drugs may suppress LH, for example pharmacological doses of corticosteroids. Hirsutism, balding or acne strongly suggest an alternative diagnosis of polycystic ovary syndrome. The examination should include weight and height, body hair

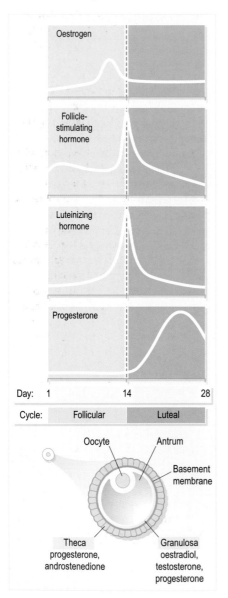

Fig. 1 **The menstrual cycle.**
The graphs show the serum hormone levels during the cycle. The development of the primordial follicle into a dominant follicle is shown. The antrum is filled with fluid. The granulosa and theca are layers of cells making sex steroids in response to luteinizing hormone and follicle-stimulating hormone stimulation.

Table 1 **Classification of causes of amenorrhoea**	
Class	**Cause**
Physiological	Pregnancy, breast-feeding, menopause
Hypogonadotrophic hypogonadism	Weight loss, stress, exercise, pituitary or hypothalamic diseases, drugs
Ovarian defects	Turner syndrome, premature ovarian failure
Uterine or genital pathology	Developmental, acquired

distribution and body shape. Short stature may indicate GH deficiency in patients with pituitary disease. A lack of body hair may indicate complete androgen resistance (p. 34–35). Body shape may suggest a functioning pituitary lesion such as Cushing's disease. Abnormal elbow-carrying angles and other skeletal abnormalities may indicate chromosomal disorders such as Turner syndrome (p. 43). The visual field and ocular movements should be examined for mass effects of a pituitary tumour. The smell should be tested for Kallmann syndrome (much less common in females as this is usually an X-linked recessive disorder).

An examination of the breasts and genitals are essential. Vaginal examinations will reveal developmental abnormalities such as an imperforate hymen. The lack of a cervix can also be detected clinically.

Investigations

A limited number of tests will yield considerable information but should be performed once pregnancy has been excluded:

- serum progesterone (in luteal phase)
- serum oestradiol
- serum LH/FSH
- serum prolactin
- serum testosterone
- thyroid function.

If the LH/FSH levels are high:

- karyotype
- pelvic ultrasound.

If the LH/FSH are low or normal:

- basal pituitary function
- magnetic resonance imaging (MRI) of pituitary or hypothalamus.

Menopause

Basic concepts

Menopause is physiological ovarian failure with loss of oocytes and follicles (atresia) and a consequent decline in ovarian sex steroid production. The average age of menopause is 50 years, with a broad variation ranging between 44 and 56 years of age. The increasing human lifespan means that the proportion of menopausal females is rising and is projected to reach 40% by 2025. The loss of ovarian steroids includes ovarian androgens, androstenedione and testosterone. Adrenal steroids, including androstenedione, are unable to compensate for this loss.

Symptoms and signs

Symptoms
Symptoms are very varied and will include some of the following:

- amenorrhoea
- flushing
- vaginal dryness
- poor libido
- labile mood
- depression
- headache
- insomnia
- pain on intercourse (dyspareunia)
- musculoskeletal aches
- joint stiffness.

The most common symptom is often flushing (called flashes in the USA). This is caused by vasodilatation in the skin, with a rise in skin temperature and sweating. The flushes are often felt in the upper body, head and neck, but also occur all over the body. They may occur multiple times a day. Flushing occurs because of oestrogen deficiency and is seen in any hypogonadism where there has previously been some sex hormone exposure. It is not specific to the menopause. Menstrual irregularity and intermittent flushing may precede amenorrhoea by several months or years; the interval leading up to menopause is called the *climacteric*. Symptoms such as loss of libido are partly related to loss of ovarian androgens.

Signs
The breast and external genitalia may show signs of regression. The vaginal walls lack secretions. There may be postmenopausal osteoporotic fractures.

Management
The aims of treatment are to alleviate symptoms and prevent postmenopausal fractures. The treatment should be bespoke and adjusted to the symptoms and end organ risks of individual patients. It is no longer appropriate to recommend one type of treatment, such as full hormone replacement therapy (HRT) for all patients with menopause. Unfortunately, full HRT is associated with increased risks (Table 2). The risk

of endometrial cancer can be reduced by opposing oestrogens with progesterones. Bile cholesterol is increased in oestrogen-treated women and this worsens gall bladder disease. Some patients may still prefer full HRT if they have severe symptoms or advancing osteoporosis. A dual energy X-ray absorptiometry (DEXA) scan to assess bone density is a useful guide to treatment priorities.

Instead of full HRT, other strategies are available (Table 3). Partial oestrogens may be used. Tibolone is a molecule that is converted into three weak metabolites: an oestrogen, a progesterone and an androgen. This may partly alleviate symptoms and benefits bone while not stimulating the breast. Raloxifene is a selective oestrogen receptor modifying drug with partial oestrogen actions. It may benefit bones. Patients with cardiovascular disease, hyperlipidaemia or bone disease may need specific treatment with a hydroxymethylglutaryl-conzyme A (HMG CoA) reductase inhibitor (statin) or a bisphosphonate. Alternative sources of oestrogen, for example plant or phytooestrogens, are sometimes used. However, they are poorly absorbed and contain complex mixtures of chemicals. Some contain flavones, implicated in goitrogenesis.

Table 2 Risks and benefits of hormone replacement therapy

Benefits	Risks
Relief of symptoms (e.g. flushing)	Breast cancer
Improvement of postmenopausal osteoporosis	Endometrial cancer
	Cardiovascular disease
	Gall stones

Table 3 Treatment strategies for menopause

Treatments	Indications
Oestrogen patches with progesterones	Severe symptoms, osteoporosis
Tibolone or raloxifene	Symptoms, osteoporosis, osteopenia
Statins	Hyperlipidaemia
Local oestrogen creams	Vaginal dryness, dyspareunia
Nocturnal oral progesterone	Night-time flushing
Clonidine	Flushing
Bisphosphonates	Osteoporosis
Calcium supplements	Prevention of osteoporosis, osteopenia
Testosterone implants or gels	Poor libido, fatigue

Female Hypogonadism

- The main manifestation of hypogonadism is menstrual abnormality.
- First exclude pregnancy.
- Weight-related amenorrhoea is a common cause of hypogonadotrophic hypogonadism.
- Flushing is caused by oestrogen deficiency.
- Examination may reveal genital or uterine pathology.

Polycystic ovary syndrome

Basic concepts

Polycystic ovary syndrome (PCOS) is a poorly named syndrome of unknown aetiology. The features are symptoms and biochemical evidence of an excess of male hormones. The origin of excess androgens may be from the adrenal or ovary or both. Enzyme defects in the sex steroid synthetic pathway have been suggested, but only found in a handful of patients. Although the aetiology is unknown, there is evidence that PCOS is part of an insulin resistance spectrum of diseases, including type 2 diabetes mellitus. There is some link to low birthweight, familial occurrence and the use of the anticonvulsant valproate. An important principle is to separate the PCOS from the isolated appearance of polycystic ovaries on pelvic ultrasound because 20% of women have ultrasound appearances of polycystic ovaries, yet only 5% of these women will have the signs and symptoms of PCOS.

There appear to be several subtypes of PCOS, with some patients being overweight and insulin resistant, some with low weights, some with coexistent hyperprolactinaemia and those treated with valproate.

Symptoms and signs

The onset of symptoms peaks between 15 and 25 years of age and include:

- hirsutism
- infertility
- oligomenorrhoea
- amenorrhoea
- capital hair loss
- acne
- recurrent miscarriage (disputed).

Hirsutism often affects the face and other areas of male distribution (Fig. 1). The presence of obesity and acanthosis nigricans indicate insulin resistance (Fig. 2). Obesity is often associated with increased subcutaneous fat and this may result in striae over the limbs (Fig. 3), in contrast to the central abdominal striae of Cushing's syndrome. However, the presence of striae should still trigger investigations to exclude Cushing's syndrome.

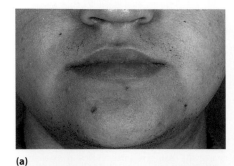

(a)

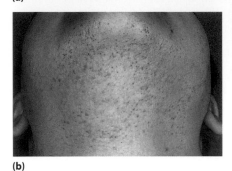

(b)

Fig. 1 **Hirsutism of the face (a) and chin (b).**

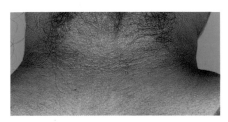

Fig. 2 **Acanthosis nigricans over skin creases on the back of the neck**

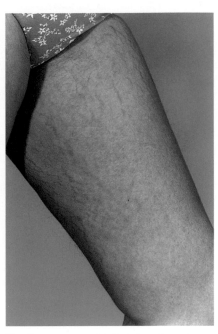

Fig. 3 **Striae over the thigh in polycystic ovary syndrome.** Note the extension of hirsutism from the pubic region.

Investigations

The biochemical assessment aims to confirm the abnormal androgen levels, test for associated risks and exclude other differential diagnoses (Table 1). A 9 a.m. blood sample on day 21 of the cycle is the simplest screening test. Androstenedione is the most commonly elevated androgen and does not vary significantly during the normal menstrual cycle.

The main associated condition is insulin resistance; this is conveniently assessed by measuring a paired fasting glucose and serum insulin. An index of insulin resistance can be obtained from these values by several computer programs (HOMA or QUICKI). The fasting glucose and glucose tolerance tests are occasionally abnormal.

Management

There is no cure. However effective control is available. The management is specifically adapted to the symptoms and needs of the patient and usually requires courses of 2 years' duration to be fully effective. Management options include:

increase oestrogen
- ethinylestradiol (Dianette) plus cyproterone acetate
- oral contraceptive pill

reduce androgen production
- weight loss/metformin
- reverse circadian prednisolone

block androgen action

Table 1 **Biochemical abnormalities in polycystic ovary syndrome**	
Test	**Characteristic**
LH/FSH	LH is 2–3-fold higher than FSH
Oestradiol	Usually normal
Progesterone	Usually low
Androstenedione	High in 80% of patients
Testosterone	Mildly elevated or normal
DHEA	Mildly elevated or normal
SHBG	Often low
17-Hydroxyprogesterone	Normal
Cortisol	Normal
Prolactin	High in 30%

- finasteride
- physical controls of hirsutism (e.g. laser)
- topical ornithine decarboxylase inhibitor (eflornithine).

Hirutism is effectively treated by increasing oestrogens and blocking androgens, with best results seen in the second year of treatment. The most convenient preparation is an oral contraceptive pill that contains a small dose of cyproterone acetate (a progesterone and androgen-receptor blocker). Some oral contraceptive pills contain progesterones that are artificially derived from androgens and may exacerbate hirsutism. In severe hirsutism, a higher dose of cyproterone acetate may be used with the oral contraceptive pill. Finasteride is also effective and blocks the conversion of testosterone to dihydrotestosterone by the tissue-specific 5-alpha-reductase enzyme. All drugs that block male hormone action may feminize a male fetus. Patients must not fall pregnant while taking these drugs and should stop 3 months before attempting conception. Improvement in hirsutism can be assessed by photography, but a scoring system (Ferriman–Gallway) has aslo been described.

Lack of ovulation requires treatment to suppress androgen levels. This may be achieved by lowering nocturnal adrenocorticotrophic hormone (ACTH) stimulation of the adrenals with reverse circadian rhythm prednisolone (Fig. 4) or with metformin. These regimens are safe but unlicenced and they require specialist supervision.

Weight loss is essential in overweight infertile patients and should probably be the only initial treatment goal in patients over 100 kg in body weight. Clomifene alone is relatively unsuccessful in inducing ovulation, but may be useful in combination with metformin or reverse circadian rhythm prednisolone.

Surgical treatments such as ovarian diathermy or wedge resection have been advocated; however, formal evidence of benefit is lacking and pelvic adhesions may be a complication.

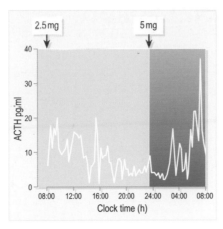

Fig. 4 **Reverse circadian rhythm prednisolone is taken to suppress noctural adrenocorticotrophic hormone (ACTH) secretion (shading).** The white line shows normal serum ACTH variation over a day. The dose of prednisolone is indicated in boxes above the graph, with arrows indicating the time of ingestion. A small morning dose prevents hypoadrenalism. Corticosteroid side-effects are not seen as endogenous adrenal steroids (including androgens) are switched off.

Differential diagnosis of polycystic ovary syndrome

Several rare but treatable conditions may mimic PCOS and should be excluded:

- congenital adrenal hyperplasia
- hypogonadotrophic hypogonadism
- Cushing's disease
- adrenal tumour secreting androgens
- ovarian tumour secreting androgens.

Congenital adrenal hyperplasia is the commonest differential diagnosis (p. 31). The late-onset form of congenital adrenal hyperplasia is about 20 times rarer than PCOS. Many patients have polycystic ovaries on pelvic ultrasound. The diagnosis is based on elevated

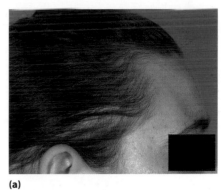

(a)

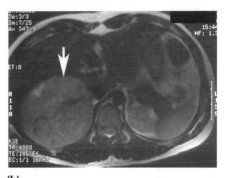

(b)

Fig. 5 A young woman presenting with hirsutism and temporal recession of capital hair (a), was found to have very high serum testosterone levels from a virilizing right adrenocortical carcinoma (b), see arrow on magnetic resonance image.

serum 17-hydroxyprogesterone levels. Lifelong treatment may be needed and there is, rarely, a risk of hypoadrenalism at times of physical stress. The condition is transmitted to fetus and children. Hypogonadotrophic hypogonadism is identified by low serum oestradiol levels. Cushing's disease is rare but the management differs radically. Adrenal and ovarian tumours are often marked by very high levels of serum testosterone (Fig. 5).

Polycystic ovary syndrome

- Polycystic ovaries on pelvic ultrasound do not necessarily mean PCOS.
- The aetiology is unknown but may be related to insulin resistance.
- PCOS is very common and there is no cure.
- A biochemical assessment of androgens is needed.
- There are some important differential diagnoses.
- There are multiple methods of control depending on symptoms.
- Prolonged treatment is needed for hirsutism.
- Associated metabolic problems should be treated.

Infertility and ovarian failure

The probability of pregnancy for a normal couple having intercourse in a single menstrual cycle is approximately 30%. Infertility is said to be present when conception has not occurred after 1 year of unprotected intercourse. Infertility can be divided into four types: female causes, male causes, combined causes and unknown. The endocrine causes of female infertility act to inhibit ovulation and are found in about 15% of cases.

Endocrine disorders in male infertility are much less frequent (Table 1); however, adequate intratesticular testosterone levels are needed for normal germ cell maturation. Oligospermic men rarely present with endocrine-related symptoms as Leydig cells can function and produce testosterone independently of the germ cells. The role of mild or subclinical varicocoeles in infertility is controversial, and their repair does not appear to restore fertility. However, clinically severe varicocoeles should probably be repaired surgically. Obstruction to the vas deferens and hypogonadotrophic hypogonadism are the most treatable causes.

Clinical assessment
The timing of menses and sexual intercourse should be documented.

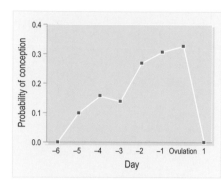

Fig. 1 **Timing of intercourse and the probability of conception.** Adapted from Wilcox et al 1995. Timing of sexual intercourse in relation to ovulation. NEJM 333:1517–21.

This may be charted by the couple. Conception is optimal in the 48 hours leading up to ovulation (Fig. 1). A history of irregular menstruation suggests lack of ovulation. A history of pelvic inflammation, pelvic surgery or severe peritonitis may indicate tubal adhesions. A full general and vaginal examination should be performed. The male history should include testicular pain, infections or trauma. The testes should be examined. The sense of smell should be assessed, particularly in patients with hypogonadotrophic hypogonadism.

Investigations
The priorities are to assess ovulation and check adequate sperm production (Table 2). Ovulation is best tested by serum progesterone level of > 30 nmol/L (10 ng/mL) on day 21 of the cycle. Home kits are available that test the urine for the LH surge, which occurs about 24 hours prior to ovulation.

A seminal analysis should be performed within an hour of a fresh sample produced by masturbation (Table 3). The traditional criterion for a normal sperm concentration is

Table 3 **Seminal analysis**		
	Subfertile	**Fertile**
Concentration (× 10⁶/mL)	< 13.5	> 48
Motility (% motile)	< 32	> 63
Morphology (% normal)	< 9	> 12

20×10^6/mL, but lower values are seen in about 25% of fertile men. Furthermore, there is a substantial overlap between the seminal analysis results from fertile and subfertile men. When the sperm count is subnormal, the male should avoid activities that increase the temperature of the testes and should wear boxer shorts and take showers rather than baths. If there are no sperm in the seminal sample, a testicular biopsy may be needed to assess whether germ cells are present.

If ovulation and the seminal analysis are normal, then a gynaecology opinion is required to assess tubal patency, pelvic diseases, immunological compatibility and consider in vitro fertilization. If an antisperm antibody is found in the female, then the use of a condom for 3 months may lower the titre and allow a somewhat increased rate of conception. Many couples are ultimately offered in vitro fertilization.

Management of endocrine causes of infertility
The simplest condition to treat is prolactinoma, with 80% of women achieving a pregnancy within three menstrual cycles after starting dopamine-agonist treatment (p. 18–19). The longest experience is with bromocriptine, but cabergoline is also effective and probably safe for the fetus. All patients should have an assessment of tumour size, because some experience swelling of the prolactinoma after coming off dopamine-agonists during the pregnancy. Patients with macoprolactinomas are at the highest risk of regrowth of the tumour and bromocriptine may have to be continued through the pregnancy. Polycystic ovary syndrome is discussed on p. 40–41.

Endocrine-aspects of gonadal stimulation
Artificial gonadotrophins are administered to stimulate the development of ovarian follicles for in

Table 1 **Causes of male infertility**	
Cause	**Percentage**
Idiopathic	42
Varicocoele	39
Cryptorchidism	6
Obstruction	5
Viral orchitis	2
Incorrect coital technique	2
Klinefelter syndrome	2
Hypogonadotrophic hypogonadism	0.8
Immotile sperm	0.6
Radiation/chemotherapy	0.2

Table 2 **Investigations in infertility**	
Female (day 21 blood sample)	**Male**
Thyroxine and thyroid-stimulating hormone	Seminal analysis
LH/FSH	LH/FSH
Oestradiol	Oestradiol
Progesterone	Sex hormone binding globulin
Prolactin	Prolactin
Testosterone	Testosterone
Androstenedione	
DHEA	

vitro fertilization. At the same time, endogenous gonadotrophins are suppressed by use of LH-releasing hormone (LHRH) agonists. Once developed, follicles are harvested by needle aspiration. The main risk is ovarian hyperstimulation syndrome, where the ovarian enlargement and excessive follicle development lead to pelvic pain and peritoneal and pelvic fluid. The situation is usually monitored by regular ultrasound and serum oestradiol measurements. Gonadotrophin treatment is interrupted if ovarian follicles or serum oestradiol levels are excessive.

Stimulation of sperm production is also used in males with hypogonadotrophic hypogonadism. The prognosis for recovery of sperm counts is good in men who have achieved a spontaneous puberty but later acquired hypogonadotrophic hypogonadism. Unfortunately, the prognosis is worse in men who failed to enter puberty spontaneously. There is no evidence that a pharmacologically induced puberty improves this prognosis. The main side-effect of gonadotrophin therapy in males is an excessive secretion of oestradiol from the testes, resulting in gynaecomastia. In addition to producing testosterone, the Leydig cells increase the amount and proportion of oestradiol in response to supraphysiological gonadotrophins.

Turner syndrome

Turner syndrome is one of the commonest chromosomal disorders, occurring in approximately 1:2500 live female births. There is a loss of one of the X chromosomes and the commonest karyotype is 45XO. The classical features are gonadal dysgenesis, short stature and skeletal abnormalities (Table 4; Figs 2 and 3). Gonadal dysgenesis is caused by accelerated atresia of ovarian follicles so that ovarian failure occurs by the time of puberty. Some patients may retain some ovarian function at puberty, with premature ovarian failure later on. There is relative growth hormone deficiency and the adult height is less than 150 cm.

Patients should have an echocardiogram, ultrasound of the kidneys and a DEXA bone densitometry scan. The treatment includes oestradiol and progesterone replacement. The replacement should be started at low doses and slowly increased in patients

Table 4 Clinical features of Turner syndrome	
System	**Features**
Gonadal dysgenesis	Primary or secondary amenorrhoea, absent puberty, immature secondary sex characteristics
Skeletal	Short stature, skeletal abnormalities, lymphoedema, short webbed neck, short 4th metacarpal, shield-like chest wall, fish-like mouth
Cardiac	Aortic valve lesions, aortic coarctation
Kidney	Horseshoe kidney
Bone structure	Osteoporosis
Autoimmune diseases	Thyroid disease, diabetes mellitus

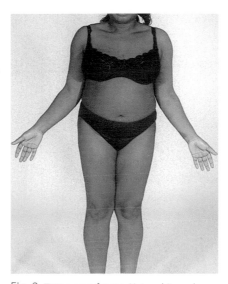

Fig. 2 **Turner syndrome.** Note cubitus valgus and short neck. The height was 148 cm.

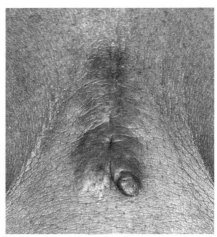

Fig. 3 **Patients with Turner syndrome are vulnerable to keloid.**

who have not had any ovarian development. The immediate introduction of standard doses may cause side-effects. Growth hormone replacement improves height and continues to be of benefit after induction of puberty.

Premature ovarian failure

Premature ovarian failure is defined as occurring below the age of 40 years.

- iatrogenic: surgery, chemotherapy or radiotherapy
- primary : part of the spectrum of organ-specific autoimmune diseases
- chromosomal abnormalities

- resistant ovary syndrome: can be reversed.

The symptoms are the same as normal menopause. The spontaneous causes are usually untreatable and the ovarian failure irreversible. A donated ovum may be used for in vitro fertilization and implantation to achieve pregnancy. The exception is the resistant ovary syndrome. Follicles are present in ovarian biopsy specimens but these fail to respond to LH and FSH. Suppression of LH and FSH for 6 months may restore follicle sensitivity. Consequently, ovarian biopsy may be offered to patients with premature ovarian failure who wish for pregnancy, provided they are counselled about the rarity of resistant ovary syndrome.

Infertility and ovarian failure

- Endocrine disorders affect a minority of infertile couples.
- Endocrine factors are more common in female infertility.
- Conception is most likely to occur in the 48 hours leading up to ovulation.
- Seminal analysis should be performed on a fresh sample.
- Ovarian hyperstimulation syndrome is a serious risk of gonadotrophin treatment.
- Turner syndrome is a chromosomal abnormality leading to premature ovarian failure.

Endocrine pancreas

The pancreatic islets of Langerhans contain four main cell types: B-cells secrete *insulin*, A-cells secrete *glucagon*, D-cells secrete *somatostatin* and PP cells secrete *pancreatic polypeptide* (the function of which is unknown). Tumours of the pancreas can arise from all cell types. Many tumours oversecrete chromogranin A which may be a useful tumour marker.

Insulinomas

The insulinoma is a rare B-cell neoplasm of the pancreatic islet that oversecretes insulin: 10% are malignant and 10% are familial. The main familial cause is multiple endocrine neoplasia type I (p. 48). Sporadic insulinomas occur at a median age of 50 years, whereas familial tumours occur at a median age of 25 years.

Symptoms and signs
Symptoms include:

- sweating
- palpitations
- weakness
- visual abnormalities
- confusion
- aggressive behaviour
- coma
- amnesia
- convulsions
- focal neurology

The classical presentation of insulinoma is with fasting hypoglycaemia, generally 4–5 hours after food intake. The symptoms of hypoglycaemia are non-specific and vary considerably between patients. Fasting hypoglycaemia is often misdiagnosed, for example, as a neurological disorder such as epilepsy. Conversely, many patients without fasting hypoglycaemia or insulinomas will have symptoms during fasting that are relieved by food intake. Rarely, insulinomas can present with postprandial hypoglycaemia.

Investigations
A blood sugar analysis during symptoms is the most valuable test. The key diagnostic criteria are known as *Whipple's triad*:

1. Appropriate symptoms (see above)
2. Documented hypoglycaemia (blood sugar < 2.2 mmol/L (40 mg/dL))

3. Symptom relief from appropriate therapy (sugar should cause relief of symptoms within a half hour).

The first clue is often from a fingerprick capillary blood tested on a portable analyser by nursing or paramedical staff. These are not accurate in the hypoglycaemic range, so a venous plasma sample should be taken immediately in an antiglycolytic-containing (fluoride oxalate) bottle and analysed urgently. A serum sample should also the taken for insulin, C-peptide and sulphonylurea levels. Intravenous glucose should then be given to the patient. The reversal of symptoms is very rapid.

Tests in insulinoma include:

- plasma glucose, low in any cause of hypoglycaemia
- serum insulin, also high in patients given exogenous insulin
- C-peptide, only made from endogenous insulin
- sulphonylurea, stimulates endogenous insulin
- 72 hour fast (supervised) to reproduce hypoglycaemia.
- magnetic resonance or CT imaging of the pancreas.

In specialist centres, the diagnosis is often confirmed by a supervised fast lasting up to 72-hours. MRI is very useful at localizing lesions, but only after the diagnosis is biochemically secure. Care should be taken in patients with multiple lesions because not all may be functioning as insulinomas, and sometimes the largest lesion is not the culprit. Insulinomas are usually < 2 cm in diameter (Fig. 1). Endoscopic ultrasound may also be needed to localize small tumours.

Other causes of hypoglycaemia are:

- artefact (e.g. delay in analysis of serum sample)
- early diabetes mellitus (postprandial)
- drugs (sulphonylureas, insulin)
- alcohol
- surgery to upper gut (postprandial)
- starvation
- adrenal failure
- galactosaemia (children)
- hereditary fructose intolerance (children)

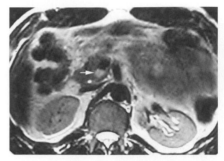

Fig. 1 **An insulinoma in the uncinate process (arrow) shown on a T$_2$-weighted magnetic resonance scan.** The patient presented with convulsions.

- non-B cell hypoglycaemia (insulin-like growth factor-2 production from mesenchymal tumours).

Management
Initial management is to give intravenous dextrose. Diazoxide blocks insulin release and is useful before surgical treatment. Definitive treatment is by local resection of the insulinoma. If the lesion is difficult to find, or if it is not resectable, long-term diazoxide treatment may be required.

Gastrinomas

Gastrinomas are rare neoplasms of the endocrine pancreas or the G cells of the duodenal or gastric mucosa: 60% are malignant and 30% are familial. They oversecrete the gut hormone gastrin, which stimulates acid release from the stomach. Multiple endocrine neoplasia type I is the main familial cause.

Symptoms and signs
The clinical syndrome caused by gastrin oversecretion is also known as Zollinger–Ellison syndrome. Features are:

- multiple peptic ulcers
- recurrent peptic ulcers
- gastrointestinal haemorrhage
- steatorrhoea
- diarrhoea.

Investigations
The fasting plasma gastrin is usually elevated but may be only mildly raised. The differential diagnosis of an elevated gastrin level is:

- proton pump inhibitors
- H$_2$-receptor antagonists

- gastritis
- upper gut surgery.

Increased gastric acid should be confirmed by pH studies. Patients should have stopped H_2-receptor blockers for 1 week and proton pump inhibitors for 3 weeks prior to testing serum gastrin. CT or MRI may show the tumour. Classically the tumour is located in the gastrinoma triangle (Fig. 2). Radiolabelled octreotide scanning may also be useful in localizing disease (Fig. 3).

Management
Patients will require high doses of proton pump inhibitors to prevent gastric acid production and peptic ulcers. Surgical resection may be curative. Metastatic disease may be very indolent and may respond slowly to chemotherapy. Octreotide treatment

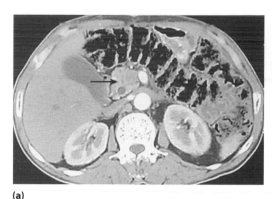

(a)   (b)

Fig. 3 **Locating a gastrinoma.** (a) A gastrinoma in the head of the pancreas (arrowed). (b) Binding of radiolabelled octreotide allows the mass to be seen in saggital view.

may reduce gastrin secretion from unresectable tumours.

Other islet cell tumours

These include:

- Non-functioning islet cell tumours
- VIPomas
- Glucagonomas

VIPomas produce high levels of vasoactive intestinal polypeptide which classically presents with watery diarrhoea, hypokalaemia and alkalosis. Patients may produce several litres per day of watery diarrhoea, thereby loosing potassium and bicarbonate. VIP also causes vasodilation and patients may have flushing and low blood pressure during attacks.

Glucagonomas over-secrete glucagon and the classical presentation is a rash called necrolytic migratory erythema, diabetes mellitus and venous

thrombosis. Necrolytic migratory erythema spreads over the groin and perineum and is initially red, but may blister and form crusts (Fig. 4, p. 77). Most tumours are malignant with metastases detectable at the time of diagnosis.

Management
Hormonal oversecretion is often easier to control than the tumour bulk. Somatostatin – analogues or steroids often help hormonal symptoms. Surgical debulking is often valuable. High doses of radioactively-labelled meta-iodobenzylguanidine or octreotide may give hormonal control if taken up by the tumour, but only a minority of patients respond with a tumour size reduction. Palliative chemotherapy with 5-fluorouracil and streptozotocin or lomustine is usually well tolerated.

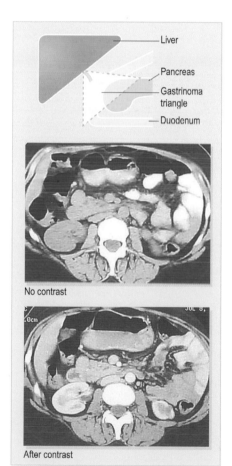

Liver

Pancreas

Gastrinoma triangle

Duodenum

No contrast

After contrast

Fig. 2 **The gastrinoma triangle is marked by the porta hepatitis, the junction of the second and third parts of the duodenum and the border between the head and neck of the pancreas.** The computed tomographic scan shows a gastrinoma (thin arrow) lying on the second part of the duodenum (thick arrow) in the gastrinoma triangle.

Endocrine pancreas

Insulinoma
- Blood glucose should be tested in any patient with acute neurological presentations.
- Fasting hypoglycaemia is a blood glucose of < 2.2 mmol/L (40 mg/dL).
- Treatment is by giving 50 mL dextrose 50% intravenous after blood sugar sample.
- Confirm the diagnosis biochemically before scanning.

Gastrinoma
- Rare neoplasms of the endocrine pancreas or the G cells of the duodenal or gastric mucosa.
- Oversecrete the gut hormone gastrin; clinical syndrome is known as Zollinger–Ellison syndrome.
- Multiple endocrine neoplasia type I is the main familial cause.

Calcium and bone: basic concepts

Calcium homeostasis

The two main concepts in calcium homeostasis are the maintenance of calcium and phosphate homeostasis in serum and the bone remodelling system. The main acute regulator of serum calcium homeostasis is parathyroid hormone (PTH) (Table 1). PTH secretion from the parathyroid glands is stimulated by hypocalcaemia and inhibited by hypercalcaemia (Fig. 1). PTH acts acutely at bone and kidney to mobilize calcium from the bone and increase resorption of calcium from the kidney: 99% of body calcium is stored in bone. Adequate dietary calcium is essential (approximately 800 mg daily) and is often not achieved. About 50% of circulating calcium is free or ionized and is the physiologically active fraction (Box 1). A second hormone, vitamin D, is important in the long-term control of serum calcium levels.

The bone remodelling unit

Bone remodelling is the gradual physiological turnover of the skeleton, at a rate of about 1% per year. The bone remodelling unit is a balance between osteoblasts and osteoclasts (Fig. 2). Osteoblast cells lay down new extracellular bone matrix and add calcium to the matrix (mineralization of bone). Osteoclast cells produce acids and proteases on their surfaces thereby

Table 1 **Actions of parathyroid hormone**	
Organ	**Effect**
High levels in bone	Bone resorption, calcium released
Low, intermittent levels in bone	Osteoblast activation
Kidney	Increased calcium resorption from tubules, reduced phosphate resorption from tubules, increased 1,25-vitamin D production
Gut	Increased calcium absorption via 1,25-vitamin D

Box 1 *Measuring serum calcium*

Principle: 50% of calcium is protein bound, usually to albumin. The total calcium level must be corrected depending on the albumin level.

Method: To derive the corrected calcium from total calcium, add 0.02 mmol/L to serum calcium for each 1 g/L that serum albumin is below 40 g/L. Conversely, subtract from serum calcium if albumin is above 40 g/L.

In the USA, where measurements are commonly given as mg/dL: add 1 mg/dL to serum calcium for each 1 g/dL that serum albumin is below 4 g/dL.

Notes. Normal ionized calcium is 1.2 mmol/L and can be estimated on blood gas analysers; in myeloma, high levels of calcium-binding paraproteins may elevate total serum calcium.

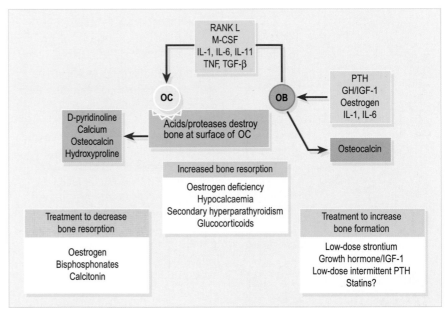

Fig. 2 **The bone remodelling unit.** PTH, parathyroid hormone; OC, osteoclasts; OB, osteoblasts; RANK L, receptor activator of nuclear factor κB ligand; M-CSF, macrophage colony-stimulating factor; IL, interleukin; TNF, tumour necrosis factor; TGF, transforming growth factor; GH, growth hormone; IGF-1, insulin-like growth factor-1.

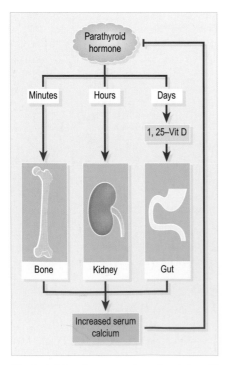

Fig. 1 **Calcium homeostasis and parathyroid hormone feedback.**

resorbing bone. Osteoclast action leads to a shift of calcium from the bone to the circulation; increased bone resorption occurs in:

- oestrogen deficiency
- hyperparathyroidism
- glucocorticoids
- hypocalcaemia.

PTH has effects on the bone remodelling unit, primarily acting through the osteoblast. In response to high levels of PTH, the osteoblasts are inhibited and release intermediate compounds that stimulate osteoclasts. Low and intermittent levels of PTH stimulate the osteoblast, but not the osteoclast, resulting in net formation of bone.

Other hormones

Vitamin D metabolites increase gut absorption of calcium and phosphate. They are required for the development and maintenance of mineralized bone (p. 51). *Calcitonin* is a peptide hormone secreted by the C cells of the thyroid. The physiological role is uncertain. There is no bone disease associated with calcitonin deficiency (for example, after total thyroidectomy). However, pharmacological doses of calcitonin inhibit osteoclasts and reduce bone resorption and serum calcium. This is useful in Paget disease (see below). PTH-related peptide is a peptide hormone that is secreted at high levels by some human carcinomas, particularly squamous cell lung cancers. It has actions similar to PTH and is a cause of hypercalcaemia. It may have physiological functions in the human fetus, but no significant endocrine actions in the human.

Paget disease

Pathogenesis
Paget disease is a classical disease of bone remodelling. It is of unknown aetiology and is particularly prevalent in the British Isles, affecting about 3% of the population. The pathogenesis involves an overactivity of osteoclasts, leading to lysis of bone. The damaged area is replaced with a highly vascular fibrous tissue. Later, an intense sclerotic reaction develops because of the high osteoblast activity. This is associated with disorganized bone formation.

Symptoms and signs
Many patients are asymptomatic. However, the commonest clinical presentation is pain; other clinical features are:

- bone deformity
- pathological fractures
- deafness
- other nerve compression.

Complications may be:

- sarcomas (rare)
- high-output cardiac failure (rare)

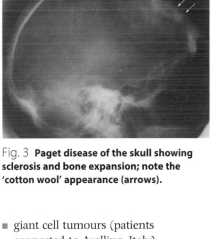

Fig. 3 **Paget disease of the skull showing sclerosis and bone expansion; note the 'cotton wool' appearance (arrows).**

- giant cell tumours (patients connected to Avellino, Italy).

The pain is dull, constant and present at night, but may be worse with movement or exertion. The disease is confined to one bone in about 25% of patients on isotope bone scanning, but usually affects several bones. The most commonly affected regions are the skull, vertebrae, sacrum and femur. The bone isoform of serum alkaline phosphatase is usually elevated. Plain radiographs show the characteristic chaotic mixture of bone lysis and sclerosis (Fig. 3). A characteristic feature is expansion of the bone. Small partial fractures (microfractures) are seen and indicate a risk of complete pathological fractures. The distribution of the disease is best shown by areas of intense uptake on an isotope bone scan (Figs 4 and 5).

Management
Bisphosphonates are the most effective treatment. Modern variants selectively inhibit osteoclasts. Patients with severe

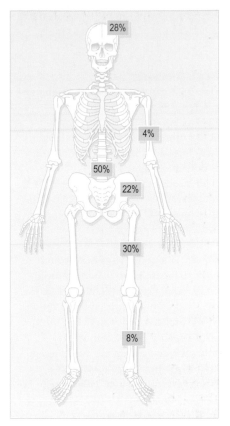

Fig. 5 **The frequency of Paget disease in the skeleton.**

manifestations may require repeated cycles of intravenous compounds. Salmon calcitonin is also effective at relieving symptoms of bone pain and reducing osteoclast activity. Orthopaedic surgery may be required, particularly for unstable fractures or fractures of the hip. Surgery may be complicated by severe bleeding from highly vascular bone.

Calcium and bone

- Parathyroid hormone is the main acute regulator of calcium homeostasis.
- Calcium is stored in bones.
- Calcium in diet is often inadequate.
- Bone is constantly remodelled.
- Osteoblasts lay down bone.
- Osteoclasts resorb bone.

Paget disease
- Paget disease is common and involves abnormal bone remodelling.
- The main symptom is pain.
- Radiographs show chaotic, expanded bone.
- Isotope bone scanning is the most sensitive test.
- Serum alkaline phosphatase may be raised.
- Treatment is with bisphosphonates and calcitonin.

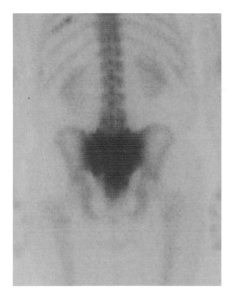

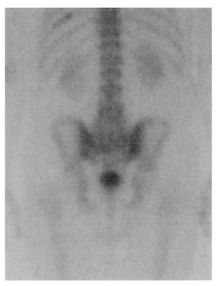

(a)   (b)

Fig. 4 **Isotope bone scans in Paget disease.** (a) Posterior scan of the sacrum. (b) The same patient after treatment.

Hypercalcaemia

Basic concepts

Hyperparathyroidism and malignancy represent 90% of the causes of hypercalcaemia (Table 1). Hyperparathyroidism is often long-standing and commonly detected by routine biochemical testing, rather than by specific symptoms (see below). Malignancy-associated hypercalcaemia may be caused by bone lysis by cytokines or metastases in patients with myeloma, lymphoma or breast cancer. The underlying disease and bone metastases are usually clinically and radiologically evident. Humoral hypercalcaemia is caused by secretion of PTH-related peptide (PTHrP) from solid tumours, most commonly squamous, renal, bladder, ovarian and breast carcinomas. A subtype of lymphoma, associated with human T-cell leukaemia virus (HTLV-1) infections, and neuroendocrine tumours may also secrete PTHrP. The biochemistry of PTHrP hypercalcaemia is similar to primary hyperparathyroidism (see below), except the serum PTH is undetectable. Hypercalcaemia may also be a consequence of increased 1,25-hydroxyvitamin D conversion in granulomas, for example in sarcoidosis (Fig. 1).

Symptoms and signs

Serum calcium is filtered in the urine and, at high levels, acts as an osmotic diuretic. Urinary symptoms tend to occur early in the evolution of the disease and include:

- polyuria
- nocturia
- polydipsia

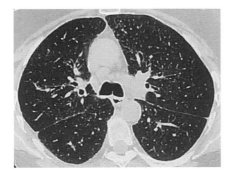

Fig. 1 **Sarcoidosis nodules in the lung in a patient with hypercalcaemia caused by increased 1,25-hydroxyvitamin D production in granulomas.**

Table 1 Causes of hypercalcaemia

	Cause
Hyperparathyroidism	Primary
Malignancy	Myeloma, haematological malignancies, multiple bone metastases
Humeral	PTH-related peptide secreted from solid tumours and some lymphomas
Hypocalciuric hypercalcaemia	Familial benign
Vitamin D excess	Intoxication, sarcoidosis
High bone resorption	Drugs (thiazides), vitamin A intoxication, immobilization, thyrotoxicosis
Renal failure	Tertiary hyperparathyroidism, vitamin D intoxication, milk-alkali syndrome

- dehydration
- renal stones
- renal failure.

When serum calcium levels are higher, abdominal and general symptoms occur:

- constipation
- abdominal pain
- lethargy
- confusion
- coma

Very high serum calcium levels (as in parathyroid storm) may lead to cardiorespiratory failure and coma, particularly if the patient is dehydrated.

Investigations

The diagnostic approach to hypercalcaemia requires an accurate assessment of serum PTH levels, in addition to clinical and radiological tests:

- full clinical examination, including skin, mouth, lymph nodes, breasts, perineum
- full blood count and erythrocyte sedimentation rate
- serum urea and electrolytes, liver function tests, calcium, phosphate, bicarbonate
- serum PTH
- serum protein electrophoresis
- thyroxine and thyroid-stimulating hormone
- 24-hour urine for calcium, phosphate
- chest X-ray.

The following should also be considered:

- serum angiotensin-converting enzyme measurements for sarcoidosis
- computed tomography (CT) of chest, abdomen and pelvis.

PTH has a half life of about 5 minutes in serum and should be rapidly centrifuged at 4°C and frozen. Serum PTH may also be misleadingly high if the sample is taken soon after an infusion of bisphosphonates or a rapid fall in calcium. The sample for PTH is best taken before any treatment is started.

High doses of corticosteroids rapidly reverse hypercalcaemia in vitamin D excess and in some malignancies. This has been used as a diagnostic and therapeutic trial (e.g. hydrocortisone 120 mg orally daily for 10 days, measuring serum calcium every 3 days).

Hyperparathyroidism

Primary hyperparathyroidism may be caused by a single adenoma, multiple adenomas, hyperplasia or carcinoma. Single adenoma is the commonest aetiology. There are several genetic causes, usually associated with multiple adenomas (Table 2 and Fig. 2). Secondary hyperparathyroidism is a response to hypocalcaemia and hyperphosphataemia of renal failure. Tertiary hyperparathyroidism occurs in

Table 2 Genetic diseases causing hyperparathyroidism

Genetic disease	Consequence
Multiple endocrine neoplasia type I	Hyperparathyroidism, pancreatic islet tumour, pituitary tumour, chest/gastric carcinoid
Multiple endocrine neoplasia type II	Medullary thyroid cancer, phaeochromocytoma, hyperparathyroidism
Hyperparathyroidism and jaw tumour syndrome	Hyperparathyroidism, concreting fibromas of jaw (Fig. 2)

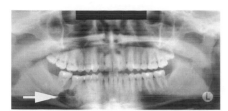

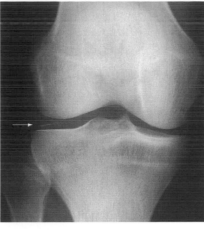

Fig. 2 **A concreting fibroma (arrow) in the mandible of a patient with familial hyperparathyroidism and jaw tumour syndrome.**

Fig. 3 **Chondrocalcinosis (arrow) in a patient with pseudogout.**

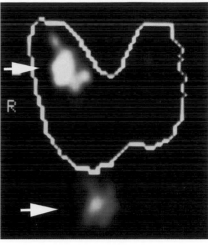

Fig. 4 **Isotope parathyroid scan with sestamibi showing two adenomas in the right upper and lower positions in a patient with multiple endocrine neoplasia type I.**

severe long-standing secondary hyperparathyroidism when hyperplastic nodules become autonomous, causing hypercalcaemia.

An important differential diagnosis to consider is familial benign hypocalciuric hypercalcaemia. This genetic disorder is caused by inactivating mutations of the calcium-sensing receptor gene. There is insensitivity of cells to high calcium levels and patients have few symptoms. The biochemical picture is similar to primary hyperparathyroidism, except the urinary calcium is very low, and family members also have hypercalcaemia. The main risk is of unnecessary parathyroidectomy, which fails to cure the condition.

The surgical anatomy of the parathyroids is that they lie behind the thyroid gland, two behind the right and two behind the left. The lower parathyroids share a common embryology with the thymus and may be found in the anterior mediastinum. More than four parathyroids occur in about 5% of individuals.

Symptoms and signs
Presentation is usually between 50 and 70 years of age. Approximately 50% will have no symptoms and so most patients will be identified on routine screening tests. The surgical tradition is that hyperparathyroidism causes problems with bones, stones, moans and groans:

- symptoms of hypercalcaemia (see above)
- depression, fatigue
- muscle weakness
- peptic ulcer
- pancreatitis
- renal stones and colic
- fractures
- pseudogout (Fig. 3)
- hypertension
- corneal calcification.

Investigations
The serum PTH is either high or in the upper half of the normal range. If the serum PTH is low, another diagnosis, or an artefact of the PTH measurement, should be considered. The main problem is localizing the site of disease. Ultrasound, CT and magnetic resonance imaging (MRI) may reveal a mass behind the thyroid. Isotope scanning with sestamibi is useful provided there is no thyroid nodularity (Fig. 4). Venous catheterization of neck and mediastinal veins for PTH levels may be useful in patients where other tests have given conflicting results.

Management
Hydration must always be maintained with intravenous saline during intercurrent illness or if kept nil by mouth. This will prevent severe hypercalcaemia as a complication of dehydration. In severe hypercalcaemia (> 3.5 mmol/L), treatment should start with intravenous saline to correct dehydration and compensate for polyuria. Bisphosphonates should only be used once the volume status is normal. The definitive treatment is surgical exploration of the neck. If there is a single adenoma, it is removed and the remaining parathyroids may be inspected and marked, but left behind. It is usual to attempt a total parathyroidectomy in all patients with multiple adenomas, hyperplasia, genetic causes or parathyroid carcinoma.

Indications for surgical treatment include:

- symptoms
- young age
- serum calcium > 3 mmol/L
- urine calcium > 10 mmol/L
- osteoporosis
- renal calcification/stones.

Most patients will require calcium supplements and vitamin D analogue treatment if parathyroidectomy is successful. If parathyroidectomy fails to cure hypercalcaemia, a diagnosis of familial benign hypocalciuric hypercalcaemia should be reconsidered. A calcium-sensing receptor agonist (Cinacalcet) may be used to control hyperparathyroidism if surgical treatment is unsuccessful.

Hypercalcaemia

- In hypercalcaemia, 90% of patients have hyperparathyroidism or malignancy.
- Hyperparathyroidism is often long standing.
- Polyuria and nocturia are common.
- Dehydration must be avoided.
- PTH is measured before treatment is started.
- Patients must be rehydrated before taking bisphosphonates.

Hypocalcaemia

The commonest causes of hypocalcaemia are vitamin D deficiency and surgical hypoparathyroidism (Table 1). Hypocalcaemia is made worse by low serum magnesium, high serum potassium or alkalosis. Hypoparathyroidism is part of a spectrum of organ-specific autoimmune disease. The polyglandular autoimmune syndrome type I consists of candidiasis, Addison's disease and hypoparathyroidism. Pseudohypoparathyroidism is caused by resistance to PTH: low serum calcium and a high serum PTH are found. Such patients may have skeletal features, including short metacarpal bones (Albright hereditary osteodystrophy; Fig. 1). The condition is called pseudopseudohypoparathyroidism when only the skeletal features, and not the hypocalcaemia, are present.

Symptoms and signs

Acute presentations
Acute hypocalcaemia results in classical neuromuscular features:

- numbness, paraesthesia
- muscle cramps
- labile mood, fatigue
- carpopedal spasm (Trousseau sign; Fig. 2)
- seizures
- stridor, wheeze
- abdominal pain
- Chvostek sign
- long QT interval on electrocardiograph.

Chronic presentations
Chronic or insidious-onset hypocalcaemia may have non-specific signs, typically involving the skin. The skin may be dry or have lesions such as psoriasis or dermatitis. There may be brittle nails, coarse hair and ectopic calcification (classically in the cornea or basal ganglia).

Investigations
The following tests are needed in hypocalcaemia:

- serum calcium, phosphate and albumin
- blood count and erythrocyte sedimentation rate
- urea and electrolytes and magnesium
- liver function tests
- serum 25-hydroxyvitamin D
- serum PTH
- serum cortisol
- 24-hour urinary calcium and phosphate.

Treatment
When hypocalcaemia is chronic or mild, most patients are treated with calcium supplements to ensure adequate dietary calcium. A vitamin D analogue is often needed for surgical hypoparathyroidism (e.g. alfacalcidol (1α-hydroxycholecalciferol)). The treatment aims are to maintain serum calcium at the low end of the normal range. The 24-hour urinary calcium should not be > 5 mmol/L as there is an increased risk of renal calculi. In severe acute

Table 1	Causes of hypocalcaemia
Causes	
Hypoparathyroidism	Iatrogenic, autoimmune, sepsis, abnormal magnesium, alcohol, genetic
Vitamin D deficiency	Dietary insufficiency, insufficient sunlight
Resistance syndromes	Pseudohypoparathyroidism, vitamin D-resistant rickets
Genetic	Activating mutation of calcium-sensing receptor

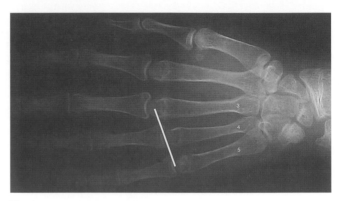

Fig. 1 **A short fourth metacarpal bone.** A line drawn from the end of the 5th to the end of the 4th metacarpal should miss the 3rd metacarpal, except when the 4th metacarpal is short, as shown.

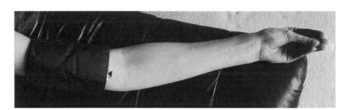

Fig. 2 **Carpopedal spasm induced during a Trousseau test.** A blood pressure cuff is inflated to 30 mmHg above systolic. The fingers and thumb cannot be easily extended by the examiner or the patient. The time to carpopedal spasm is recorded. A normal result is no spasm after 3 minutes of arterial occlusion.

Box 1 Emergency treatment of hypocalcaemia

Indication: serum calcium < 2 mmol/L *and* symptoms.
A calcium infusion 15 mg/kg is given over 4 hours in 1 litre saline.
Practical guide: volume (mL) of 10% calcium gluconate that is required is given by 1.7 × body mass (kg).

hypocalcaemia, intravenous calcium infusions may be needed (Box 1). Recombinant human PTH (teriparatide) is now available as daily subcutaneous injections.

Vitamin D deficiency

Vitamin D is a hormone synthesized in skin and activated by enzymes in the liver and kidneys (Fig. 3). Ultraviolet light converts a cholesterol metabolite into vitamin D precursors.

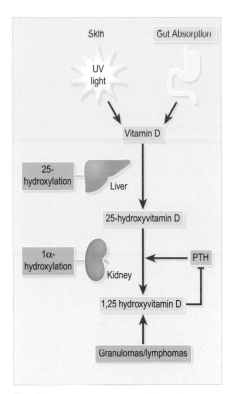

Fig. 3 **The vitamin D metabolic pathway.**

Skin production of vitamin D is low or undetectable in winter months in residents of northern latitudes. The other source of vitamin D is diet, but only a limited number of foods contain high concentrations, e.g. fish livers or egg yolks. Risk factors for vitamin D deficiency are:

- dwelling at high latitude
- vegetarian diet
- elderly or housebound
- hospitalized or chronically ill
- upper gastrointestinal surgery
- small bowel disease
- phenytoin use
- chronic liver and renal disease.

Patients at increased risk for vitamin D deficiency include the elderly and those taking foods containing phytates (e.g. chapatis), which inhibit calcium absorption from the gut.

Actions of 1,25-hydroxyvitamin D include:

- absorption of dietary calcium and phosphate
- suppression of PTH production
- formation of bone remodeling unit.

Symptoms and signs

Muscle pains are common in adults with vitamin D deficiency and often occur in the absence of other classical features:

- muscle pain/weakness
- bone pain/deformity
- pathological fracture (Looser's zones)
- slipped epiphyses (rickets)
- waddling gait
- tiredness
- symptoms of hypocalcaemia (see above).

Muscle weakness affects proximal muscles, especially around the hips, causing the classical waddling gait. Bone deformity and fractures are caused by inadequate mineralization (calcium) of the bone matrix. Rickets occurs in children and osteomalacia in adults. Small pseudofractures or microfractures are called Looser's zones (Fig. 4).

The classical signs of rickets depend on the developmental stage of the child. Neonatal rickets affects the skull (ping-pong ball skull) and ribs with swollen epiphyses (the so-called

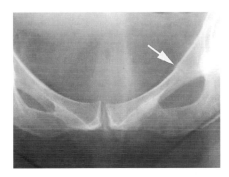

Fig. 4 **Looser zone (a microfracture) in the left superior ramus in metabolic bone disease.**

ricketic rosary). Older children may develop bow-legs or knock-knees.

Investigations

In severe disease, serum 25-hydroxyvitamin D, calcium and phosphate are low, and serum alkaline phosphatase and PTH are elevated. It is important to note that many patients with undetectable serum vitamin D have normal serum alkaline phosphatase levels. A significant minority of patients with bone biopsy-proven osteomalacia has serum 25-hydroxyvitamin D levels that are between 20–50 nmol/L.

Treatment

A number of vitamin D pharmaceuticals are available (Table 2). An oral supplement of ergocalciferol (calciferol) 800 U daily is cheap and effective in the treatment of vitamin D deficiency. A higher dose (10,000 U weekly) may be needed for patients with severe bone disease or symptoms. Treatment may be monitored clinically and by serum calcium and 25-hydroxyvitamin D levels (aim for > 50 nmol/L). Analogues that do not require hydroxylation (e.g. 1,25-hydroxyvitamin D) are often used for patients with liver or renal disease.

Table 2 **Vitamin D pharmaceuticals**	
Drug[a]	**Vitamin D form**
Ergocalciferol (calciferol)	Vitamin D_2
Cholecalciferol	Vitamin D_3
Alfacalcidol (1α-hydroxycholecalciferol)	1-Hydroxyvitamin D
Calcitriol (1,25-dihydroxycholecalciferol)	1,25-Dihydroxyvitamin D
[a]US name given in parentheses.	

Hypocalcaemia

- The commonest causes of hypocalcaemia are vitamin D deficiency and surgical hypoparathyroidism.
- Vitamin D deficiency can result from lack of sunlight and from dietary factors.
- Muscle pain and weakness are common in vitamin D deficiency.
- Serum calcium and alkaline phosphatase are often normal in vitamin D deficiency.
- Treatment with oral ergocalciferol is effective and cheap.
- Vitamin D analogues are usually needed in hypoparathyroidism, renal or liver disease.

Osteoporosis

Basic concepts

Osteoporosis is a decreased bone mass. Increasing holes or spaces develop between the matrix and the bone is more porous. The density of the bone is, therefore, decreased. The remaining bone matrix has normal mineralization (calcium), unlike in *osteomalacia*, where mineralization of bone matrix is reduced (p. 51). The consequence of reduced bone mass is fragile bones and fractures. Osteoporotic fractures will affect about 40% of females and 13% of males.

The term *osteopenia* has several uses: as a general term in radiology for radiolucent bones, without quantification of severity; and as a definition on bone densitometry scans (DEXA: dual energy X-ray absorptiometry) as an intermediate stage of bone density before osteoporosis (see below).

Osteoporosis is caused by many conditions and is, therefore, a description and not a diagnosis:

- increasing age
- oestrogen or testosterone deficiency
- excessive alcohol
- low calcium intake
- vitamin D deficiency.

Other major risk factors are:

- family history
- immobilization
- heparin
- smoking
- chronic obstructive airway disease
- endocrine diseases: glucocorticoid excess, thyrotoxicosis, hyperparathyroidism, hyperprolactinaemia
- gastrointestinal disease
- bone marrow/connective tissue diseases.

Most patients have several factors that have increased the risk of osteoporosis. In female patients, postmenopausal osteoporosis is the commonest. Smoking, lack of exercise, excessive alcohol use, a lack of calcium in the diet and a family history may coexist. Many risk factors are reversible; for example, vitamin D deficiency should always be excluded.

The underlying pathophysiology is an imbalance in the bone remodelling unit (Fig. 2, p. 46). Thus, bone resorption is abnormally increased compared with bone formation. Bone formation normally increases at puberty and peaks at about 20 years of age. A failure to achieve peak bone mass because of hypogonadism or delayed puberty is a rare mechanism of osteoporosis.

Symptoms and signs

There are no symptoms until fractures develop. A fracture with minimal trauma indicates osteoporosis or osteopenia:

- fall from own height
- falls of < 13 cm
- deceleration from speeds less than a run.

Fractures can occur in several sites:

- vertebral spine (most frequently)
- femoral neck
- wrist
- ankle.

The patient may notice a progressive loss of height, with a stooped posture. A full menstrual and drug history is required. Heparin may cause increased bone resorption within a few weeks of treatment.

Investigations

Investigations are aimed at identifying reversible risks:

- blood count and erythrocyte sedimentation rate
- serum tests of renal function
- serum calcium
- serum 25-hydroxyvitamin D
- serum PTH
- serum testosterone or oestradiol
- serum thyroxine and thyroid-stimulating hormone
- serum prolactin
- 24-hour urine calcium and phosphate
- DEXA bone mineral densitometry.

Plain radiographs are not sufficiently sensitive to identify osteoporosis before fractures have occurred. DEXA is a common method of quantifying bone density. It is predictive of future fractures (Table 1). A DEXA scan is of less use in a patient who has already sustained a low-energy fracture as many of these patients will require treatment.

Management

Risk factors such as smoking, alcohol use or immobility should be explained to the patient. Pharmacological therapy is based on treatment to reduce bone resorption or to increase bone formation (Table 2). Most patients with established osteoporosis will benefit from calcium and vitamin D and a bisphosphonate. Oral bisphosphonates may cause gastrointestinal side-effects and highly potent intravenous bisphosphonates that act over a year are available at

Table 1 **Assessing bone mineral densitometry with DEXA**

	Comments
Advantages	Predicts fracture risk
	Monitors response to treatments
Pitfalls	Misleading in bones with fractures/sclerosis
	Does not indicate underlying cause
	Different machines may give different results
Interpretation	Compares bone density to young adult population (T-scores)
WHO criteria are based on T-scores	Normal 0 to −1
	Osteopenia −1 to −2.5
	Osteoporosis −2.5 or below

Table 2 **Managements for osteoporosis**

Management	Comment
Identify and remove cause (if possible)	Examples are vitamin D deficiency, gastrointestinal disease
Reduce risk factors	Smoking, alcohol use, immobility
Treatment to reduce bone resorption	Oestrogen, bisphosphonates, calcitonin
Treatments to increase bone formation	Low dose PTH, HMG-CoA reductase inhibitors (statins), low-dose fluoride, growth hormone/IGF-1, strontium
HMG-CoA, 3-hydroxy-3-methylglutaryl conezyme A; IGF, insulin-like growth factor.	

Box 1 Treatment of postmenopausal osteoporosis

Counsel against smoking and alcohol.
Calcium 1000 mg and vitamin D 800 IU (in the UK, calcium plus ergocalciferol, two tablets daily), taken daily.
Oral bisphosphonate, taken daily or weekly.
Intravenous bisphosphonate (if oral bisphosphonate not tolerated); zoledronate can be given once a year.
Oestrogen replacement (e.g. tibolone), see p. 38–39.
Repeat assessment by DEXA bone mineral density in 12–24 months.

similar cost. Treatment of postmenopausal osteoporosis (Box 1) has become increasingly common. The use of oestrogens in postmenopausal osteoporosis requires an assessment of cardiovascular and breast cancer risks, since these are increased by full hormone replacement therapy (p. 38–39).

Patients with osteopenia on bone densitometry are also at increased fracture risk; they may also need treatment, particularly if a risk factor continues to be present. One common situation is the use of glucocorticoids. The most effective treatment for patients taking glucocorticoids is a potent bisphosphonate, such as alendronic acid or risedronate. Calcium and vitamin D supplements alone may suffice for patients taking very low doses of glucocorticoids and who have normal bone density.

Patients treated for osteoporosis should be reviewed clinically within a few weeks of starting treatments to ensure compliance and a lack of side-effects. A biochemical assessment of calcium, electrolytes and renal and liver function is performed. The next follow-up assessment can be after one year of treatment, at which point a DEXA bone mineral density scan is repeated to ensure that the condition is not worsening. Subsequent clinical and bone mineral density assessments can be at two-yearly intervals, since changes in bone density are slow. In patients with risk factors for osteopenia or osteoporosis, hip and lumbar spine bone density measurement are preferred as these are the sites that are most vulnerable to clinically significant fractures and that respond to therapy. Heel or forearm bone density measurements may be more appropriate in patients at low risk as these techniques are cheaper and simpler to perform.

Osteoporotic fractures
The main sites of fracture are the wrists, hips and vertebrae. A hip fracture carries the worst prognosis and is treated surgically, followed by mobilization and therapy to prevent further fractures. Acute vertebral compression fractures (Fig. 1) have traditionally been treated medically, with bedrest, analgesia and sometimes calcitonin.

Percutaneous techniques now allow rapid relief of pain and patient mobilization. Percutaneous vertebroplasty involves the introduction of a needle under radiological guidance into the compressed vertebral body, followed by the injection of an acrylic cement. Percutaneous kyphoplasty involves inserting a balloon via a needle into the vertebral body, inflating the collapsed bone and then fixing it with acrylic cement (Fig. 2). About 80% of patients are mobile within 24-hours of such procedures and patient satisfaction with the treatment is very high. The risks are embolization, cord compression and potential for worsening the fracture risks in other vertebral bodies (particularly in glucocorticoid osteoporosis).

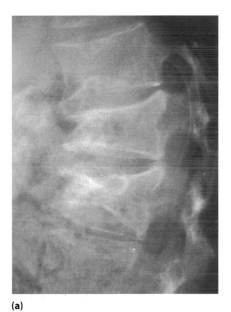
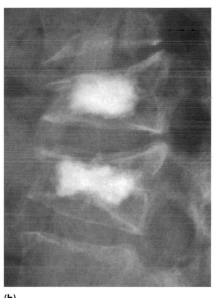

(a)   (b)

Fig. 1 **Vertebral compression fractures due to osteoporosis (a) may be treated by percutaneous balloon kyphoplasty.** A balloon catheter is introduced into the vertebral body and inflated, followed by an injection of cement (b). This treatment is particularly effective at controlling pain. (Courtesy of Mr John Yeh.)

Osteoporosis

- Osteoporosis is decreased bone mass and presents with fragility fractures.
- The commonest risk factors are age, sex hormone deficiency, alcohol and smoking.
- Always exclude vitamin D deficiency prior to treatment.
- Treatment with bisphosphonates is most effective at reducing fracture risk.
- Monitor with DEXA bone mineral density scans.

Diabetes mellitus

What is diabetes?

Background

The features of the disease that we now call diabetes mellitus, or simply 'diabetes', were first identified by the Ancient Egyptians (Fig. 1). Subsequently, other authors over the centuries have described the classic features of increased urine and blood sugar and thirst, the critical role of insulin, and the pancreas as its source. More recently, the two- and three-dimensional structures of insulin have been elucidated and the molecule synthesized (Table 1).

What is diabetes?

Diabetes mellitus is a chronic disorder caused by high blood glucose; it is often referred to simply as 'diabetes'. Since we all have glucose in our blood, it follows that there is a threshold level that defines diabetes. This definition has varied over the years and can presently be determined by either a raised fasting glucose or a raised glucose following oral glucose challenge (Table 2). Diabetes mellitus may be primary or secondary to another disease. Primary forms are:

- type 1 (insulin-dependent diabetes mellitus; IDDM)
- type 2 (non-insulin-dependent diabetes mellitus; NIDDM)
  - non-obese
  - obese
- malnutrition-related (rare, in tropics)
- gestational (occurs for first time in pregnancy).

Although secondary diabetes mellitus (Table 3) accounts for barely 1–2% of all new cases, it is important to recognize because it often needs different therapy.

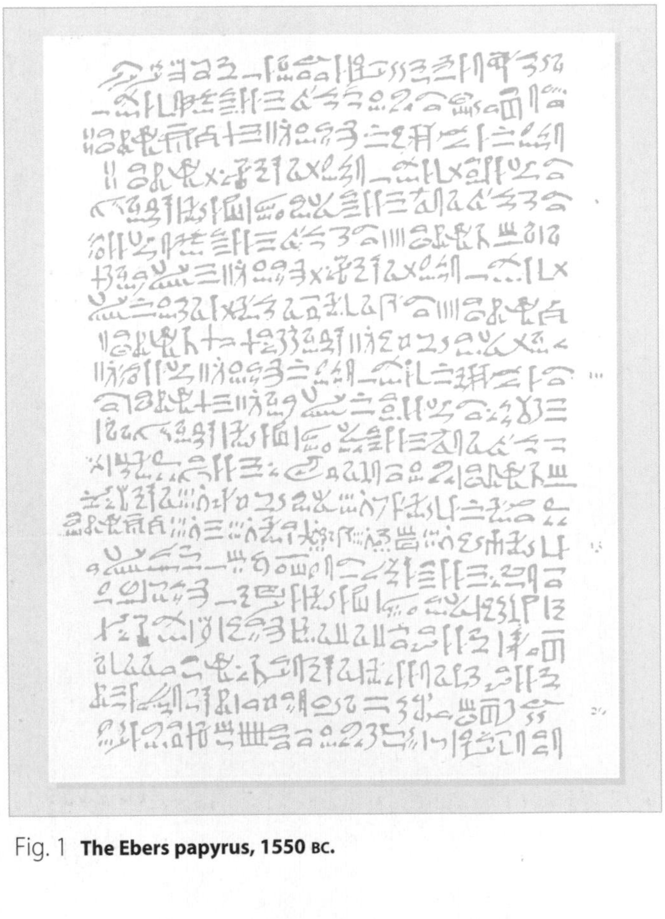

Table 1 Historical milestones in diabetes mellitus

Date	Source	Observation
1550 BC	Egyptian papyrus (Fig. 2.29.1)	Excessive amounts of urine
1–2nd century AD	Galen (Roman), Aretaeus (Greek)	Sugary urine, excessive thirst
5th century	Susruta, Charuka (Indian)	Described sugary urine, distinguished obese and thin patients
10th century	Avicenna (Arabia)	Sugary urine; gangrene and impotence as complications
17th century	Willis (England)	Diabetic urine contains sugar
18th century	Dobson, Cawley (England)	Sugar in serum in diabetes; diabetes may follow pancreatic damage
19th century	Bernard (French)	Glucose stored as glycogen on liver; exocrine degeneration of the pancreas occurs after ligature of the pancreatic duct
19th century	Langerhans, Minkowski, von Mering (Germany)	Pancreatic islets; pancreatomy causes diabetes
20th century	Banting, Best, MacLeod, Collip (Canadian)	Discovery of insulin
20th century	Hodgekin, Sanger (England)	Structure of insulin

Table 2 Interpretation of oral glucose tolerance test

	Venous plasma glucose, mmol/L (mg/dL)	
	Fasting	120 min after 75 g glucose load
Normal	< 6.1 (110)	< 7.8 (140)
Impaired fasting glucose	≥ 6.1 (110) (110–125)	
Impaired glucose tolerance	–	7.8–11.1; (140–199)
Diabetes mellitus	> 7.0 (126)	≥ 11.1 (200)

NB: In the absence of symptoms, a diagnosis of diabetes must be confirmed by a second diagnostic test (i.e. a fasting, random, or repeat glucose tolerance test) on a separate day.

Table 3 Secondary causes of diabetes mellitus

Conditions	
Pancreatic disease	Chronic or recurrent pancreatitis, haemochromatosis
Other endocrine disease	Cushing's syndrome, acromegaly, phaeochromocytoma, glucagonoma
Drugs	Glucocorticoids, corticotrophin, diuretics, β-blockers
Abnormalities of insulin or its receptor	Insulinopathies, insulin receptor defects, circulating antireceptor antibodies
Genetic	DIDMOAD syndrome, lipoatrophic diabetes, cystic fibrosis

Type 1 and type 2 diabetes mellitus represent two distinct diseases, but clinically the distinction can sometimes be misleading and uncertain; for example, loss of insulin secretion is most severe in type 1 but may be present across the spectrum of diabetes. Less commonly, loss of insulin secretion may also be a feature of type 2. Decreased insulin sensitivity is most severe in patients with type 2 diabetes but may also be found in other types.

Clinical presentation

Patients with diabetes mellitus present with either symptoms of high plasma glucose or clinical problems resulting from

Fig. 1 **The Ebers papyrus, 1550 BC.**

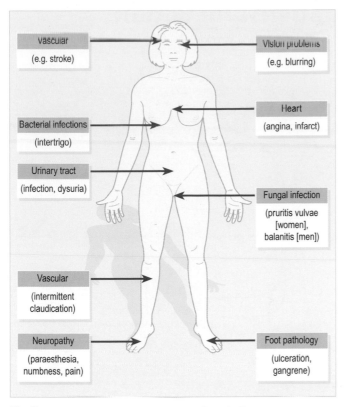

Fig. 2 **Identification of diabetes mellitus from indirect consequences.**

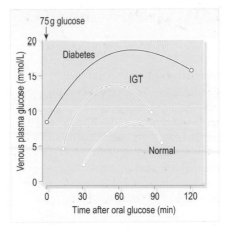

Fig. 3 **Impaired glucose tolerance (IGT) is a state between normal and diabetes.**

the high glucose. Patients with type 1 diabetes often present with severe symptoms of hyperglycaemia. The severity of the condition may be reflected in raised blood ketone levels and weight loss. These symptoms are most often seen in children with type 1 diabetes:

- polyuria
- bedwetting
- thirst
- weight loss
- dehydration
- coma.

Older patients are often identified by symptoms not directly related to the metabolic dysfunction (Fig. 2) or by routine screening:

- insurance employment medical
- pregnancy
- population survey
- routine check in at-risk individual.

Ketoacidosis may be a presenting feature. Note that glycosuria is not diagnostic of diabetes mellitus but indicates the need for further investigations. About 1% of the population has renal glycosuria, inherited as an autosomal dominant or recessive trait associated with a low renal threshold for glucose.

The classic triad of symptoms are:

- polyuria: caused by the osmotic diuresis that results when blood glucose levels exceed the renal threshold
- thirst: caused by the resulting loss of fluid and electrolytes
- weight loss: caused by fluid depletion and the accelerated breakdown of fat and muscle secondary to insulin deficiency, so less prevalent in those with type 2 diabetes.

Clinical problems from high glucose include:

- lack of energy
- visual blurring (retinopathy or as a result of glucose-induced changes in refraction)

- fungal infections (pruritus vulvae and balanitis)
- bacterial infections (staphylococcal skin infections)
- polyneuropathy (tingling and numbness in the feet or erectile dysfunction).

Impaired glucose tolerance is a state of glucose tolerance between normal and diabetic states (Fig. 3); it can occur in both the obese and the non-obese but it does have certain associations:

- a family history of type 2 diabetes
- age
- central and total obesity
- physical inactivity
- fetal malnutrition
- ethnicity.

Subjects with impaired glucose tolerance are at risk of macrovascular disease and may already have arterial disease on presentation, including myocardial infarction and gangrene.

Diabetes mellitus

- Classical symptoms are polyuria, thirst and weight loss.
- Primary diabetes is divided into type 1 and type 2.
- Type 1 (insulin dependent) is associated with the development of ketoacidosis and is characterized by absolute deficiency of insulin.
- Type 2 (non-insulin-dependent) usually occurs in patients over 40 years of age, is associated with insulin resistance and only relative insulin deficiency; ketoacidosis does not usually occur.
- Impaired glucose tolerance is an intermediate state and carries health risks.

Glucose homeostasis and insulin action

Glucose homeostasis

To understand inappropriately high blood glucose, it is necessary to understand how the body maintains normal blood glucose between strict levels. These (using whole blood or plasma) are usually within the range 3.5–8.0 mmol/L (63–144 mg%), and invariably 2.5–11.0 mmol/L in health, despite the demands of food, fasting and exercise. Glucose homeostasis is organized predominantly in the liver, which absorbs glucose and stores it in the form of glycogen. Glucose is then released into the circulation between meals (Fig. 1). To maintain homeostasis, the rate of glucose utilization by peripheral tissues must match the rate of glucose production. The liver produces glucose, a six carbon molecule, by a process called *gluconeogenesis* (Fig. 1). This process involves the assembly of two 3-carbon molecules into the 6-carbon glucose. The 3-carbon molecules are themselves derived from breakdown of fat (glycerol), muscle glycogen (lactate) and protein (such as alanine).

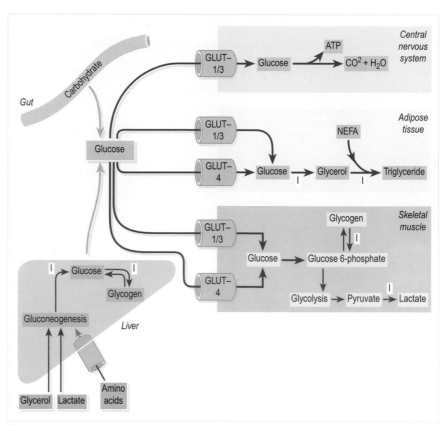

Fig. 1 **Overview of carbohydrate metabolism.** GLUT is a glucose transporter; I, indicates a site of action of insulin.

Glucose production
Approximately 200 g of glucose is produced each day. The liver produces more than 90% of this amount first from liver glycogen and second from hepatic gluconeogenesis. The remainder derives from renal gluconeogenesis.

Glucose utilization
About 200 g of glucose is utilized each day. The brain is the major consumer of glucose, using up some 100 g daily. Glucose uptake by the brain is obligatory and is not dependent on insulin. The glucose used is oxidized to carbon dioxide and water. In other tissues, notably muscle and fat, glucose uptake is variable, depending on the state of the tissue: that is, it is facultative. Glucose taken up by muscle is stored as glycogen or broken down to lactate, which re-enters the circulation where it is an important substrate for hepatic gluconeogenesis. Glucose taken up by fat tissue is used as a source of energy and as a substrate for triglyceride synthesis.

Insulin synthesis, secretion and action
Insulin is the key hormone involved in both the storage and the controlled release of chemical energy available from food. It is a peptide of 51 amino acid residues (Fig. 2) and is synthesized in the beta cells of the pancreatic islets. It is initially synthesized as a precursor, which undergoes proteolytic cleavage to give insulin and C-peptide (connecting peptide). These are stored in granules and cosecreted in equimolar amounts into the portal circulation.

Insulin enters the liver, which is its prime target organ, but C-peptide is only partially extracted by the liver. As a result, levels of C-peptide are used as an index of insulin secretion. The production and release of insulin from the beta cell, including the cellular events triggering the release of insulin from secretory granules, is illustrated in (Fig. 3). There is both a steady basal level of insulin secretion and a response to increased blood glucose levels. About 50% of secreted insulin is extracted and degraded in the liver; the residue is broken down by the kidneys.

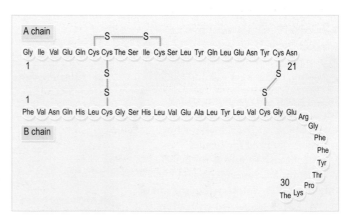

Fig. 2 **Primary structure (amino acid sequence) of human insulin.** S–S indicates a disulphide bond.

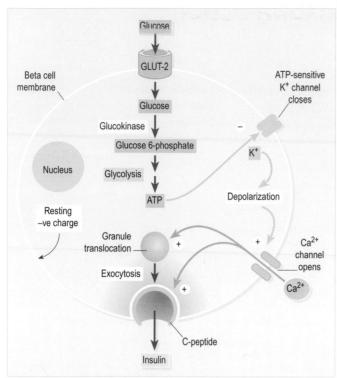

Fig. 3 **Insulin synthesis is coupled to its secretion.** GLUT is a glucose transporter.

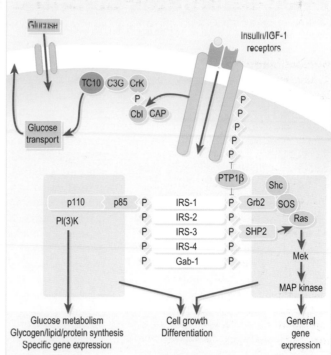

Fig. 4 **The insulin receptor and signal transduction in insulin action.**

Insulin is a major regulator of metabolism, although its actions are modified by other hormones. The effect of counter-regulatory hormones (glucagon, adrenaline, cortisol and growth hormone) is to cause greater production of glucose from the liver and less utilization of glucose in fat and muscle for a given level of insulin. The action of insulin differs in the fasting and postprandial state. During fasting, the body's energy requirements are largely met by fatty-acid oxidation. After food intake, insulin secretion peaks rapidly by secretion from the pancreatic islets into the portal circulation. The circulating insulin levels lower the threshold for glucose entry into cells.

The insulin receptor

The insulin receptor is a large glycoprotein that is expressed on the cell membrane of many cells. The receptor is a dimer with two α-subunits, which include the binding sites for insulin, and two β-subunits, which traverse the cell membrane (Fig. 4). When insulin binds to the α-subunits, there is a conformational change in the β-subunits. This conformational change results in activation of an intracellular tyrosine kinase and initiation of a cascade of intracellular responses. One such response is the migration

of the GLUT-4 glucose transporter to the cell surface; here it acts as a glucose shuttle and increases transport of glucose into the cell. The insulin-receptor complex is then internalized by the cell; insulin is degraded, and the receptor is recycled to the cell surface. Insulin has a broad range of actions (Table 1; Fig. 5).

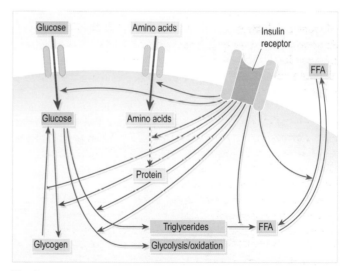

Fig. 5 **The regulation of metabolism by insulin.**

Table 1	**Physiological actions of insulin**
Type of action	**Effects**
Metabolic action	Suppression of hepatic glucose production
	Stimulation of glucose uptake by muscle and adipose tissue
	Promotion of glucose storage as glycogen
	Suppression of lipolysis and hepatic ketogenesis
	Regulation of protein turnover
	Effects on electrolyte balance
Other longer-term actions	Regulation of growth and development (in utero and post-utero)
	Regulation of expression of certain genes

Glucose homeostasis and insulin action

- Gluconeogenesis in the liver produces glucose from fat, glycogen and protein.
- Insulin in the key regulator of glucose homeostasis.
- Insulin action is predominant after a meal.
- Insulin receptors mediate the broad range of action of insulin.

Type 1 diabetes mellitus

Epidemiology

Type 1 diabetes mellitus is caused by severe insulin deficiency leading to insulin-dependent diabetes. There are several variants:

- type 1A: autoimmune
- type 1B: subacute pancreatitis in Japan
- LADA: latent autoimmune diabetes in adults.

In Western countries, almost all patients have the immune-mediated form of the disease. Type 1 diabetes is the second-commonest disease of childhood after asthma. The peak incidence is reached around the time of puberty, but it can present at any age. The highest rates of type 1A diabetes in the world are in Finland and other northern European countries (Fig. 1), and the island of Sardinia, which for unknown reasons has the second highest rate in the world. The incidence appears to be increasing in most European populations, particularly in children under the age of 5 years.

One variant of type 1 diabetes mellitus, LADA, is characterized by a slow progression to insulin deficiency.

This variant occurs in about 10% of adult patients presenting initially with non-insulin-requiring diabetes mellitus. Most of these adults will progress to insulin dependence. LADA is characterized by the presence of diabetes-associated antibodies to glutamic acid decarboxylase (GAD). Type 1B diabetes mellitus has been noted in Japanese patients. These patients progress rapidly to insulin dependence in adult life without diabetes-associated antibodies. However, increased serum amylase is found, which is consistent with a subacute pancreatitis.

Pathogenesis

Type 1 diabetes is an immune-mediated organ-specific disease. It is induced by an environmental event or events operating in a genetically susceptible individual (Fig. 2). Genetic susceptibility is polygenic (caused by the influence of multiple genes), with the greatest contribution from the histocompatability (HLA) region on the short arm of chromosome 6, a region closely involved with mounting an immune response to invading agents (Table 1). The risk of developing diabetes by age 20 years is greater with a diabetic father (3–6%) than with a diabetic mother (2–3%). The peak incidence of the disease is in adolescence but the disease can occur at any age (Fig. 3). The risks of developing diabetes mellitus are approximately 1:400 in the general population but 1:2 in an identical twin of a young diabetic

twin, 1:10 in the identical twin of an adult diabetic twin, and 1:17 in a sibling of subject with type 1 diabetes; however, it is only 1:5 if the sibling is HLA identical to the affected sibling (Table 2). The striking discordance between identical twins must be a consequence of non-genetic, probably environmental, factors. For those who present in childhood, these environmental factors probably operate in early life, even in utero. The nature of the environmental factors is unknown but candidates include:

- general factors
  - hygiene
  - parasites
  - coexisting infections (tuberculosis or malaria)
- specific factors
  - viruses (e.g. enteroviruses)
  - bacteria
  - cow's milk (through early exposure)
  - toxins.

Table 1 **HLA genotype risk classes for type 1 diabetes mellitus**	
Genetic risk for type 1	**Genotype**
High	DR3/4, DQB1 *0302
Moderate	DR4/4, DQB1 *0302
	DR3/3
	DR4/X, DQB1 *0302
	DR3/X
	DR3/4 not DQB1 *0302
	DR4/X not DQB1 *0302
	DR4/4 not DQB1 *0302
Low	DR2/4, DQB1 *0302
	DR2/4 not DQB1 *0302
	DR2/3
	DRX/X, 2/X O 2/2
	DR4*0403/X, DQB1*0302
DRX, not DR3, DR4, DR2.	

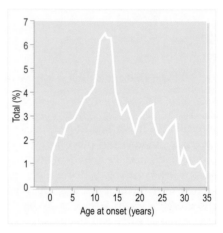

Fig. 3 **Age at onset of type 1 diabetes up to 30 years.**

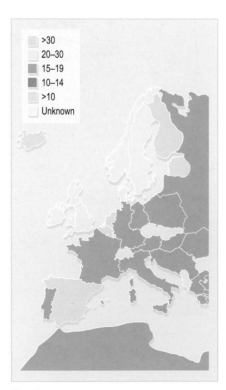

Fig. 1 **Incidence rate of type 1 diabetes (onset 0–14 years) in Europe (cases/100 000 per year).**

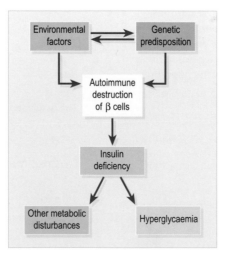

Fig. 2 **Aetiological events in type 1 diabetes.**

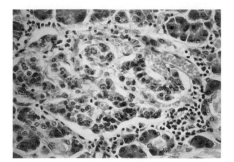

Fig. 4 **Insulitis of islet of Langerhans in a child with recent onset type 1 diabetes.**

The interaction of environmental and genetic factors leads to the induction of immune changes, including activation of T-lymphocytes and the production of autoantibodies. It is likely that the altered immune response targets the pancreatic islets; at diagnosis children show lymphocytes and macrophages surrounding and infiltrating the islets, presumably directly or indirectly destroying the insulin-secreting islet cells (Fig. 4). One model for the development of autoimmunity is shown in Figure 5. The use of autoantibodies in predicting and screening for type 1 diabetes mellitus is covered on page 66.

The evidence is that autoantibodies do not cause type 1 diabetes but instead reflect the autoimmune process which leads to the disease. Since autoantibodies can be induced at an early age, so by implication can the disease process and, since that process tends to be chronic, it follows that autoantibodies can predict the onset of

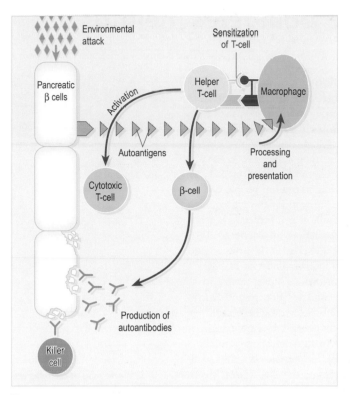

Fig. 5 **A hypothetical model showing how an environmental insult to the pancreas could lead to destruction of pancreatic beta cells by autoantibodies, killer cells and antibody-dependent complement (C) and T-cells.**

clinical disease. Some adults presenting with non-insulin requiring diabetes have diabetes-associated autoantibodies to glutamic acid decarboxylase (GAD). Such patients, mistakenly diagnosed initially with type 2 diabetes, have autoimmune non-insulin requiring diabetes designated latent autoimmune diabetes of adults (LADA). This form of autoimmune diabetes affects about

10% of recently diagnosed non-insulin requiring European adults, implying that it is more prevalent than childhood type 1 diabetes. About 90% of LADA patients progress to insulin dependence wihin 6 years, so that, rates of progression to insulin dependence apart, it is difficult to distinguish between adult-onset type 1 diabetes and LADA.

Table 2 **Family risks of developing diabetes for relatives of diabetic subjects**		
	Approximate risk (%)	
	Type 1	Type 2
Children of diabetic parents		
Diabetic father	8	? ≈ 15
Diabetic mother	2	? ≈ 15
Both parents diabetic	Up to 30	Up to 75
Siblings of diabetic patients		
Two HLA haplotypes identical	16	–
One HLA haplotype identical	9	–
No haplotypes identical	3	–
High titre diabetes associated antibodies	Up to 90	–
Any sibling	–	≈ 10
Co-twins of diabetic twins		
Identical	40	≈ 90
Non-identical	15	10

Type 1 diabetes mellitus

- Type 1 diabetes is a chronic progressive autoimmune disease.

- The incidence of type 1 diabetes is highest in children.

- Type 1 diabetes is associated with autoimmune features and includes a broad range of clinical presentations at all ages.

- Identification of autoantibodies in the general population can predict type 1 diabetes.

Type 2 diabetes mellitus

Epidemiology

Type 2 diabetes mellitus is a world-wide disease: the rate of increase is such that there is effectively a global epidemic of the disease. Most patients with diabetes mellitus have type 2 diabetes. In 1985 the World Health Organization (WHO) estimated that 30 million people had diabetes mellitus; today the estimate is above 100 million and projections are that this prevalence will double to 200 million by 2020 (Fig. 1). There is a wide variation in the prevalence of diabetes mellitus worldwide. Whilst people in developed countries, Europe and North America, have shown the highest prevalence in general, in the next 25 years those from developing countries around these industrialized zones, such as Mexico, Egypt, the Gulf States, Russia and Ukraine, will have the highest prevalence. Apart from racial factors, the prevalence of type 2 diabetes mellitus is associated with increasing age, increasing calorie intake and decreasing calorie expenditure and obesity, as well as with pregnancy, certain drug therapy and intercurrent illness. In the UK, the prevalence using WHO criteria is about 2% and in those with an affected family member about 30%. In some hunter-gatherer groups, recently exposed to the Western lifestyle, such as Pima Indians and Naruans from Micronesia, the prevalence rises towards 80%.

Genetic factors associated with type 2

Prospective studies of identical twins of a patient with type 2 diabetes mellitus indicate that they have a greater than 90% chance of developing diabetes; though cross-sectional population-based

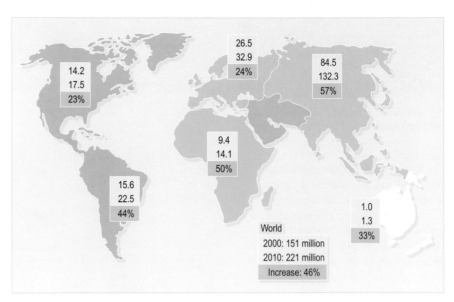

Fig. 1 **World map of diabetes mellitus frequency.** Numbers in millions for 2000, 2010 and percentage increase, respectively. (From Zimmet P, Alberti KG, Shaw J. Global and Social implications of the diabetic epidemic. Nature 414: 782–7, with permission.)

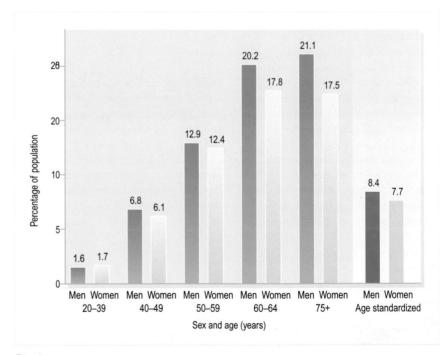

Fig. 2 **Age at onset of type 2 (adult-onset) diabetes in the USA.**

Table 1	**Main clinical characteristics of MODY subgroups**					
	HNF-4α (MODY1)	Glucokinase (MODY2)	HNF-1α (MODY3)	IPF-1 (MODY4)	HNF-1β (MODY5)	MODY-X
Frequency in a large UK series (%)	2	20	64	< 1	2	12
Penetrance of mutations at 40 years of age (%)	> 80	45 (> 90% with FPG > 6 mmol/L)	> 95	> 80	> 95	Not known
Onset of hyperglycaemia	Adolescence, early adulthood	Early childhood (from birth)	Adolescence, early adulthood	Early adulthood	Similar to HNF-1α	Uncertain
Severity of hyperglycaemia	Progressive: may become severe	Mild with little deterioration with age	Progressive; may be severe	Similar to HNF-4α	Similar to HNF-1α	Variable
Microvascular complications	Frequent	Rare	Frequent	Few data	Frequent	Variable
Pathophysiology	Beta dysfunction (glucose sensing)	Beta cell dysfunction	Beta cell dysfunction Sulphonylurea sensitive	Beta cell dysfunction	Beta cell dysfunction	Beta cell dysfunction
Other features		Reduced birth weight	Low renal threshold; sensitivity to sulphonylureas	Pancreatic agenesis in homozygotes	Renal cysts, proteinuria, renal failure	

HNF, hepatic nuclear factor; IPF, Insulin promotor factor.

studies found the risk was only 50% or less; the risk to non-identical twins or siblings is of the order of 15–25% (see Table 2, p. 61). These observations confirm a genetic component to the disease. Type 2 diabetes mellitus is a polygenic disorder, but the genes responsible remain poorly defined.

However, the genetic causes of some rare forms of type 2 diabetes have recently been determined. Decreased insulin sensitivity resulting from mutations of the insulin receptor has been described but this affects < 1% of all type 2 patients. Other insulin-resistant syndromes are associated with obesity, hyperandrogenism in women and often an area of hyperpigmented skin (ancanthosis nigricans). Individuals with some mutations or deletions of mitochondrial DNA develop type 2 diabetes mellitus or impaired glucose tolerance, in association with rare neurological syndromes.

Altered insulin action is found in rare genetic abnormalities affecting the structure of the insulin molecule. These mutant insulin molecules are associated with hyperinsulinaemia and varying degrees of glucose intolerance.

A rare variant of type 2 diabetes mellitus is referred to as 'maturity-onset diabetes of the young' (MODY). This form tends to be dominantly inherited and onset is not always in childhood. Five variants have been described. The different MODY genotypes are associated with different clinical and metabolic phenotypes (Tables 1 and 2; Fig. 3). MODY should be considered in young people presenting with a typical family history (diabetes affecting a parent and 50% expression of the disease in the family).

Environmental and other factors

The risk of type 2 diabetes mellitus and glucose intolerance is associated with low weight both at birth and at 12 months of age, and particularly in those who gain excess weight as adults. Poor nutrition early in life may impair beta cell development and function, predisposing to diabetes in later life. Low birth weight has also been shown to predispose to heart disease and hypertension in later life (Table 3).

Table 2 **A comparison of type 2 diabetes and MODY syndromes**

	Type 2 diabetes	MODY
Age of onset	Predominantly in middle to old age, but increasingly recognized in children too[a]	Childhood to young adulthood
Pathophysiology	Insulin resistance and beta cell dysfunction	Beta cell dysfunction
Role of environment	Considerable	Minimal
Associated obesity	Common	Uncommon
Inheritance	Polygenic/heterogeneous	Monogenic/autosomal dominant

Usually associated with obesity in children, and in those belonging to high-risk ethnic groups.
Sourced from Hattersley AT. *Diabetic Med* 1998; 15: 15–24.

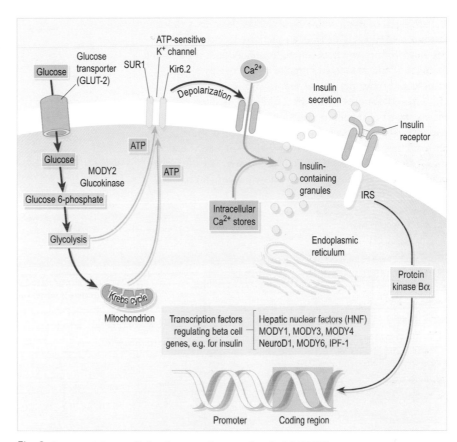

Fig. 3 **Pancreatic beta cell showing proteins associated with MODY.**

Table 3 **Determinants and risk factors for type 2 diabetes**

Type	Factors
Genetic	Genetic markers, family history, 'thrifty gene(s)'
Demographic	Demographic characteristics Sex, age, ethnicity
Behavioural and lifestyle related	Obesity (including distribution of obesity and duration) Physical inactivity Diet Stress 'Westernization, urbanization, modernization'
Metabolic determinants and intermediate risk categories	Impaired glucose tolerance Insulin resistance Pregnancy-related determinants (parity, gestational diabetes, diabetes in offspring of women with diabetes during pregnancy, intrauterine mal – or overnutrition)

Immunology

There is no evidence of immune involvement in the pathogenesis of type 2 diabetes mellitus, but about 10% of non-insulin-requiring patients have islet autoantibodies – insulinoma-related antigen (ICA) and GAD (see p. 61)–at diagnosis and are more likely to progress to insulin therapy. Such cases may have type 1 diabetes mellitus masquerading as type 2 diabetes mellitus.

Abnormalities of insulin secretion and action

Type 2 diabetes mellitus is associated with resistance to the normal actions of insulin. It is presumed that insulin can bind normally to its receptors on the surface of cells but polygenic abnormalities underlying the disease attenuate the transmission of the insulin signal within the cells, producing 'insulin resistance'. This leads to increased glucose production from the liver (owing to inadequate suppression by insulin) and inadequate uptake of glucose by skeletal muscle and other peripheral tissues (Fig. 4; see also Fig. 5, p. 59). Patients with type 2 diabetes mellitus may also have a defect of insulin production and secretion from the pancreas. However, unlike those with type 1 diabetes, patients may retain about 50% of their pancreatic beta cell mass. Almost all patients show islet amyloid deposition at autopsy, derived from a peptide known as amylin or islet amyloid polypeptide (IAPP). Its role in causation of the disease is uncertain. Abnormalities of insulin secretion develop early in the course of type 2 diabetes mellitus and in some cases are associated with potassium ion channels which are important for insulin secretion. The majority of patients manifest progressive loss of pancreatic beta cell function over several years (Fig. 5). It is not known whether this is a result of 'exhaustion' of surviving beta cells or some independent process of damage. Figure 6 shows the association of key components of the insulin resistance syndrome.

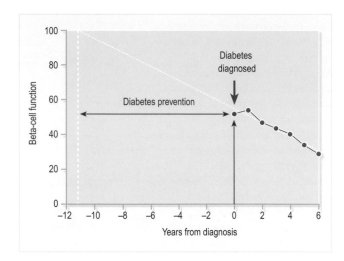

Fig. 5 **Progression of loss of insulin secretion. The period before diagnosis is when prevention could theoretically be considered.**

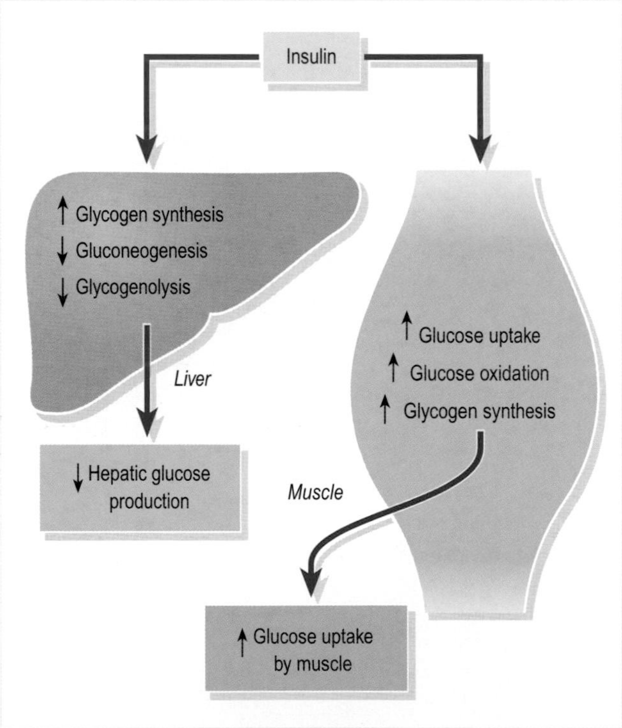

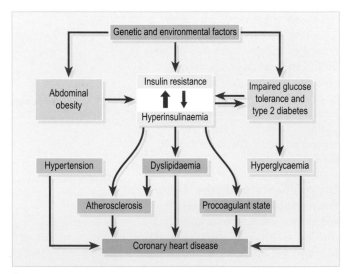

Fig. 6 **Association of key components of the insulin resistance syndrome.**

Fig. 4 **Direct actions of insulin on glucose metabolism.**

Table 1 **Definition of Metabolic Syndrome by NCEP, ATPIII: three or more of the following risk factors***	
Risk factor	**Defining level**
■ Abdominal obesity waist circumference	Men > 102 cm (> 40 in)
	Women > 88 cm (> 35 in)
■ Triglycerides	> 150 mg/dL (≥ 1.7 mmol/L)
■ HDL-cholesterol	Men < 40 mg/dL (< 1.04 mmol/L)
	Women < 50 mg/dL (< 1.29 mmol/L)
■ Blood pressure	≥ 130/≥ 85 mmHg
■ Fasting plasma glucose	≥ 110 mg/dl (≥ 6.1 mmol/L)
*3rd report of National Cholesterol Education Program (NCEP) expert panel, Adult Treatment Panel III (ATPIII). Circulation 2002; 106:3143–421.	

Causes of acquired insulin resistance

■ Glucose Toxicity
■ Lipotoxicity
■ Regional fat deposits.

Insulin resistant state may be present in 25% of the non-diabetic population, with an estimated conversion rate from an insulin resistant state to type 2 diabetes of 2–12% per year. Insulin resistance occurs more often than would be expected by chance in patients with type 2 diabetes, but also in association with hypertension, dyslipidaemia, obesity, atherosclerosis and polycystic ovary sydrome. Persistent hyperglycaemia per se can reduce insulin action by reducing insulin stimulated tyrosine kinases activity of the insulin receptor. An increase in fatty acid levels can impair both insulin secretion and insulin mediated glucose disposal and oxidation as well as increasing hepatic glucose production. Abdominal obesity, and not obesity in general, is associated with diabetes-risk. Visceral adipocytes are particularly resistant to the action of insulin. Fatty infiltration of the liver is also associated with insulin resistance and known as non-alcoholic steatohepatitis (NASH).

The metabolic syndrome

The concept that clustering of cardiovascular risk factors can occur in individuals more often than would be expected by chance led to the identification of a constellation, or syndrome, called *syndrome X, Reaven's syndrome* or the *metabolic syndrome*. The risk factors are linked in such a way that the prevalence of each factor is increased in those individuals with the other factors. Approximately 10–20% of those with type 2 diabetes mellitus have this syndrome, depending on how it is defined. The components of the metabolic syndrome are:

■ hypertension: defined as antihypertensive treatment or blood pressure > 160/90 mmHg, or both
■ dyslipidaemia: defined as elevated plasma triglyceride (≥ 1.7 mmol/L) or low high density lipoprotein (HDL) cholesterol (< 0.9 mmol/L in men; < 1.0 mmol/L in women)
■ obesity: defined as high body mass index (≥ 30 kg/m^2) or high waist–hip ratio (> 0.90 in men; > 0.85 in women)
■ microalbuminaemia: defined as overnight albumin excretion 20 µg/min.

Polycystic Ovary Syndrome

Polycystic ovary syndrome (PCOS) is probably the most common endocrine disorder in young women. The condition is associated with hirsutism, acne and problems with menstruation (oligomenorrhoea) and conception. The disorder is associated with obesity and insulin resistance and probably a higher risk of type 2 diabetes. Insulin resistance leads to hyperinsulinaemia which may stimulate ovarian androgen production by acting as a gonadotrophin. Potential therapies include metformin and thiazolidinediones, both agents used to improve insulin sensitivity in diabetes.

Type 2 diabetes mellitus

■ Type 2 diabetes is a chronic progressive disease with some retention of insulin secretion.
■ The incidence of type 2 diabetes is highest in adults.
■ Type 2 diabetes is associated with either decreased insulin secretion or insulin sensitivity or both.
■ Type 2 diabetes includes a broad range of clinical syndromes that can present at all ages.

Prevention and screening for diabetes mellitus

Criteria for testing

The occurrence of a pre-diabetic state, with changes that can be detected long before symptoms become apparent, has led to the development of criteria for testing for diabetes in asymptomatic individuals. In those over 45 years these are:

- a first-degree relative with diabetes
- overweight or obese (particularly abdominal obesity)
- impaired glucose tolerance (on previous testing)
- impaired fasting glucose
- previous gestational diabetes or large baby (≥ 4.5 kg)
- polycystic ovary syndrome
- essential hypertension
- hypertriglyceridaemia
- low HDL cholesterol
- high-risk ethnic group
- premature cardiovascular disease
- therapy with corticosteroid, high-dose thiazide, β-blocker
- primary hyperuricaemia or gout
- specific endocrinopathies (e.g. Cushing's syndrome, acromegaly, phaeochromocytoma)
- certain inherited disorders (e.g. Turner syndrome, Down syndrome).

Type 1 diabetes

Prediction

The immune changes associated with type 1 diabetes can be detected months, even years, before the clinical onset of the disease. These changes, notably the presence of autoantibodies (Fig. 1), can predict the disease; some antibodies and particularly combinations of antibodies being more predictive than others (Table 1).

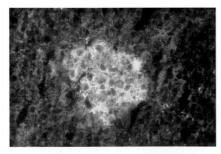

Fig. 1 **Antibody binding to islet cells.**

Table 1 **Autoantibody markers for development of type 1 diabetes**					
Antibody		Diagnostic (%)		Predictive value (%)	
	Abbreviation	Sensitivity	Specificity	First-degree relatives	General population
Islet cell antibodies	ICA	80–90	96–99	20–50	20–30
Insulin autoantibodies	IAA	40–70	99	< 50	ND
Glutamate decarboxylase	GAD	70–90	99	> 50	ND
Insulinoma-related antigen-2	1A-2	70–90	99	> 50	ND
ND, not determined.					

Screening

Autoimmune diseases are the third leading cause of morbidity and mortality in the USA, only surpassed by cancer and heart disease. Most autoimmune diseases are thought to be complex disorders involving the interaction of environmental factor(s) with more than one genetic factor. The identification of these disease-associated factors would be invaluable in predicting the risk of developing a particular autoimmune disease. However, very few have been identified and, even in those that are known, their function in pathogenesis remains uncertain. In general, autoimmune diseases are chronic disorders that develop over the course of years and are characterized by autoantibodies, which appear in the peripheral blood long before clinical symptoms. Since the presence of these autoantibodies reflects the underlying disease process, autoantibodies could be more reliable predictive markers than the presence of high-risk genes.

The feasibility of screening for autoantibodies as predictors of disease has been convincingly demonstrated in type 1 diabetes in studies involving thousands of subjects and showing that autoantibodies can predict diabetes with a degree of certainty. These autoantibodies

- can appear at an early age, even around the time of birth
- can precede the clinical onset of diabetes by some years
- can recognize some autoantigens in a manner that is more predictive than others (Table 1)
- have a positive predictive value that increases for one, two or three autoantibodies from approximately 10% to 50% and 80%, respectively, within 5 years and even higher thereafter.

The findings with autoantibodies in subjects at risk of type 1 diabetes indicate that such screening will be useful in predicting other chronic autoimmune diseases. If specific autoantibodies are predictive of disease, they can be widely used not only as part of standard laboratory work-up but also to identify subjects at risk in the immediate family. If therapeutic intervention trials are available, then antibody tests would identify those suitable for prevention therapy. With the development of high-throughput procedures and new specific and sensitive assays requiring only a few microlitres of serum, it is now feasible to consider autoantibodies as predictors of type 1 diabetes mellitus.

Type 2 diabetes mellitus

Impaired glucose tolerance (see p. 57) was defined in 1979 by the National Diabetes Data Group and the WHO and recognized then as a risk factor for type 2 diabetes mellitus. The standard definition was updated in 1985 and again in 1999 but the evidence remains that impaired glucose tolerance is a powerful predictor of progression to diabetes and is itself associated with a risk of macrovascular disease. Impaired glucose tolerance is common, affecting up to 25% of adults in UK and USA. Risk of progression to type 2 diabetes mellitus depends on a family history of diabetes mellitus, age, central and total obesity, physical inactivity, fetal maturation and ethnic origin. Impaired fasting glucose is associated with a lower risk of progression to diabetes mellitus than impaired glucose tolerance. The broad metabolic disorders associated with impaired glucose tolerance reflect those found in type 2 diabetes. Impaired glucose tolerance is an insulin-resistant state. In addition, subjects with impaired glucose tolerance have a lower insulin response to glucose challenge; this decreased response is most marked in the initial 10 minutes following glucose challenge (called the first-phase insulin response as it represents the release of insulin held in storage in the insulin-secreting islet cells). Finally, impaired glucose tolerance is associated with an increased rate of endogenous glucose production by muscles and liver.

Prevention of type 2 diabetes mellitus

Evidence from long-term lifestyle intervention trials (Table 2) suggests that lifestyle interventions are more effective in the prevention of type 2 diabetes mellitus than the drugs tested. The Finnish Diabetes Prevention Study comprised 522 middle-aged overweight subjects (172 men; 35 women) with impaired glucose tolerance who were randomly assigned to an lifestyle intervention group or a control group. The intervention involved individual counselling regarding weight loss, total fat intake, saturated fat intake, fibre intake and physical exercise. The group was followed for a mean of 3.2 years and a glucose tolerance test was performed annually. Type 2 diabetes was confirmed by a second test. Figure 2 shows the results of the trial. The conclusions drawn were:

- the risk of diabetes was reduced by 58% in the intervention group
- this risk reduction was directly linked to lifestyle changes
- those who lost 5% of their body weight had a 74% risk reduction
- those who exceeded the recommended 4 hours exercise per week had an 80% risk reduction.

These results may be expected since lifestyle intervention focuses on the

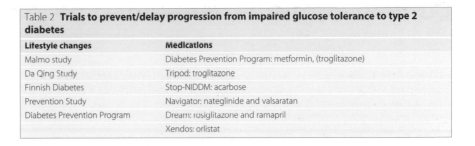

Table 2	Trials to prevent/delay progression from impaired glucose tolerance to type 2 diabetes	
Lifestyle changes	**Medications**
Malmo study	Diabetes Prevention Program: metformin, (troglitazone)
Da Qing Study	Tripod: troglitazone
Finnish Diabetes	Stop-NIDDM: acarbose
Prevention Study	Navigator: nateglinide and valsaratan
Diabetes Prevention Program	Dream: rosiglitazone and ramapril
	Xendos: orlistat

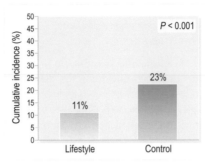

Fig. 2 **Results of Finnish prevention trial for type 2 diabetes.** The results shown are the diabetes incidence after 4 years of intervention; there was a 58% risk reduction in the group with a lifestyle intervention. (Data from Tuomilehto J, Lindstrom J, Eriksson JG 2001. Prevention of type 2 diabetes mellitus by changes in lifestyle among subjects with impaired glucose tolerance. N. Engl J Med 344:1343–50.)

pathogenic mechanisms underlying the development of type 2 diabetes mellitus, in particular factors causing insulin resistance. Theoretically, it would be possible to prevent up to 70% of type 2 diabetes in persons at increased risk if they were able to maintain normal body weight and engage in physical activity throughout their lives. More than preventing diabetes, a healthy diet and lifestyle could prevent or retard heart disease. Middle-aged subjects with impaired glucose tolerance have been successfully treated with metformin, acarbose, orlistat, troglitazone, simvastatin and angiotensin-converting enzyme inhibitors to prevent diabetes mellitus (Table 3). The task of population screening for impaired glucose tolerance is very large, but the potential for successful therapeutic intervention is also significant.

Table 3	Interventions in a diabetes prevention trial[a]
Intervention	**Reduction in the development of diabetes compared with control group (%) after 3 years**
Intensive lifestyle counselling	58
Metformin	31
Troglitazone	23 (over 10 months)[b]

[a]All eligible participants received standard lifestyle recommendations and were randomized to three treatment groups and a control group (1000 in each group).
[b]Drug stopped after 10 months.

Prevention and screening

Type 1
- Prediction of type 1 diabetes is highly accurate. Autoantibodies associated with type 1 diabetes can be detected months or years before the clinical onset of the disease.
- There is no preventative therapy at present, though intervention studies are underway.

Type 2
- Prediction is not accurate.
- Can be prevented by lifestyle or drug intervention in selected subjects.

Complications I: basic concepts

Over a period of time diabetes mellitus causes tissue damage, seen clinically as complications. Diabetes mellitus:

- shortens life expectancy by up to one third
- increases the risk of heart diease three-fold
- is the commonest single cause of limb amputations
- the commonest cause of blindness in middle-aged adults in developed countries
- the commonest cause of renal failure in middle-aged adults in developed countries.

Much of the morbidity can be prevented by good medical care, particularly control of blood glucose levels and early detection of complications.

The complications of diabetes mellitus include:

- tissue complications: largely caused by macro- and microvascular disease
- metabolic complications: hypo-and hyperglycaemia
- increased susceptibility to infections
- pregnancy-related complications
- psychosocial complications.

Macrovascular complications
Macrovascular (large vessel) disease is diffuse, affecting smaller as well as large arteries. Complications include:

- stroke
- cardiovascular disease
- renovascular disease
- peripheral vascular disease.

These are more prevalent in diabetes but are not specific to it. They may occur at a younger age in diabetic patients.

Microvascular complications
Microvascular complications are specific to diabetes mellitus but occur irrespective of the cause of the diabetes. Small blood vessels throughout the body are affected and this has particular impact on the blood supply to nerves, leading to *neuropathy*, to retina leading to retinopathy, and to the glomerulars

contributing to nephropathy. Microvascular disease has a particular clinical impact at three sites:

- retina (retinopathy)
- renal glomerulus (nephropathy)
- nerve sheaths (neuropathy).

Several factors determine the risk of developing macrovascular or microvascular disease.

- *Diabetes mellitus duration.* As with non-diabetic individuals, the risk of macrovascular disease increases with age and hence with diabetes duration. Complications tend to manifest themselves 10–20 years after diagnosis in young patients. A patient who does not develop renal disease by 30 year's postdiagnosis is unlikely to develop that complication. Patients with proteinuria, the hallmark of nephropathy, are at increased risk of macrovascular disease. The cardiovascular risk increases twofold in the presence of microalbuminuria. Retinopathy can be present at diagnosis of type 2 diabetes, probably because unrecognized diabetes existed for several years prior to diagnosis.
- *Genetic factors.* Cardiovascular disease risk is higher in diabetic women than diabetic men relative to non-diabetic individuals, as the usual cardiovascular protection in non-diabetic women is lost. Diabetic siblings of diabetic patients with renal and eye disease have a three to fivefold increased risk of the same complication whether they have type 1 or type 2 diabetes mellitus. Patients rarely develop microvascular complications if they have diabetes caused by a glucokinase polymorphism associated with raised fasting glucose but minimal postprandial hyperglycaemia.
- *Racial factors.* Some races are at higher risk of macrovascular or microvascular complications than others. For example, in the USA, the rank order of microvascular risk is Pima American Indians > Hispanic/ Mexican origin > US African origin > US European origin.

Modifiable risk factors
Five risk factors for both macrovascular and microvascular disease are modifiable and important targets of prevention therapy. These risk factors probably extend to the full range of microvascular complications:

- exercise
- hypertension
- dyslipidaemia
- smoking
- hyperglycaemia

Exercise Reduced exercise is a major risk factor in the development of type 2 diabetes. An increase in physical activity causes an improvement in both insulin sensitivity and blood glucose levels. These effects are seen before any reduction in body weight. The mechanism of improved insulin sensitivity remains unclear but possibilities include an increase in skeletal muscle blood flow, as muscle blood flow is an important determinant of glucose uptake. Exercise is associated with a reduction of risk in macrovascular disease.

Hypertension A high blood pressure is an important cause of both macrovascular and microvascular disease. Between 50–80% of patients with type 2 diabetes have hypertension (defined as > 140/90 mmHg). The prevalence of hypertension reflects the prevalence of the background population, being particularly frequent in patients of African extraction. The nature of the association between hypertension and diabetes remains unclear but it is particularly associated with obesity and insulin resistance.

Dyslipidaemia Altered lipid levels increase the risk of both macrovascular and microvascular disease in diabetes, and the risk of cardiovascular disease is greater in patients with diabetes than in non-diabetic individuals for any given cholesterol level. Type 1 diabetes is not associated with a specific lipid profile but patients with type 2 diabetes are more likely to have hypertriglyceridaemia and a low HDL-cholesterol level. Poor diabetes control,

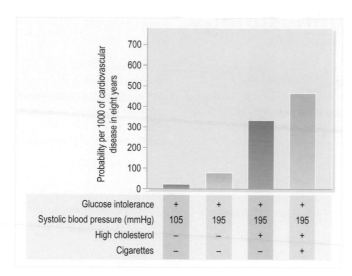

Fig. 1 **Effect of multiple risk factors on cardiovascular disease risk in a selected population with glucose intolerance.**

Glucose intolerance	+	+	+	+
Systolic blood pressure (mmHg)	105	195	195	195
High cholesterol	–	–	+	+
Cigarettes	–	–	–	+

diabetic nephropathy and treatment with beta-adrenergic receptor blockers and thiazides are each specifically associated with changes in the blood lipid profile.

Smoking Smoking increases the risk of both macrovascular disease and microvascular disease, notably nephropathy, in diabetes. About 5 million people die annually from smoking and about half of the people who smoke will die as a result of it.

Hyperglycaemia Hyperglycaemia increases the risk of both macrovascular and microvascular disease in diabetes. There is evidence that this increase in risk for both macrovascular and

microvascular disease is evident even when the glucose tolerance is only impaired. Indeed, an increased risk of macrovascular disease can even be detected in those individuals with glycated haemoglobin or blood glucose

levels at the upper end of the normal range.

Multiple risks for complications

The increased morbidity and mortality associated with type 2 diabetes mellitus have been attributed mainly to accelerated macrovascular disease, in particular cardiovascular disease, but there is also an increased risk of microvascular disease. Hyperglycaemia, hypertension, obesity and dyslipidaemia are all associated with an increased risk of macrovascular cardiovascular disease, and this effect is exaggerated in type 2 diabetes through a network of risk factors. When these risk factors occur concurrently, the aggregation is called the 'metabolic' or 'insulin resistance' syndrome (p. 64), since these conditions are all associated to a degree with insulin resistance and can precede type 2 diabetes. Such an insulin-resistant state may be present in 25% of the non-diabetic population, and in adult life approximately 2–12% per year of these individuals progress to diabetes.

Complications I: basic concepts

- Diabetes causes both macrovascular and microvascular disease.
- Unknown genetic factors play a role in complication risk.
- The risk factors for macro- and microvascular disease are similar.
- Risk factors can aggregate as in the metabolic syndrome.

Complications II: pathophysiology

Macrovascular complications

The pathogenesis of atherosclerosis, from the initial phase of leukocyte recruitment to late events such as rupture of vulnerable plaques, predominantly involves inflammatory processes including the release of inflammatory mediators. Normal vascular homeostasis is regulated by an intricately interconnected network of endothelial and smooth muscle cells. Endothelial cells act as a semi-permeable gateway, maintaining the blood in a liquid state and producing mediators that promote vascular homeostasis (notably nitric oxide and lipid factors such as prostacyclin (prostaglandin I_2)). Contraction of smooth muscle cells regulates the vascular tone of arteriolar walls, thereby determining both systolic blood pressure and peripheral blood flow. In diabetes, this intricate network is disturbed, resulting in atherogenesis. Endothelial cell dysfunction occurs early in the pathology of atherosclerosis and is common in patients with traditional risk factors – even in the absence of manifest atherosclerotic lesions. Such endothelial dysfunction predicts progression to atherosclerosis and the rate of suffering cardiovascular events.

Several markers of an inflammatory response are elevated in the peripheral blood of patients with atherosclerosis as well as in patients with type 2 diabetes mellitus. C-reactive protein is an acute-phase reactant thought to be a marker of vascular inflammation. C-reactive protein is localized within the atheromatous plaque and its expression precedes the recruitment of leukocytes at the surface of the vessel wall. Since levels of proinflammatory mediators such as C-reactive protein and fibrinogen are increased in the plasma of patients with diabetes, they may serve as markers of vascular risk.

Microvascular complications

The cause of diabetic microvascular disease is unclear, but some relevant factors are similar to those involved in macrovascular disease. An important difference is the role of hyperglycaemia, which plays a role in predisposing to macrovascular disease but is critical in the development of microvascular disease. Hyperglycaemia leads to endothelial cell damage as well as other complications. Factors associated with pathogenesis of microvascular complications include:

- hyperglycaemia
- advanced glycation end-products
- reactive oxygen species
- activation of the transcription factor NFκB
- sorbitol accumulation in cells
- activation of cell protein kinase C
- haemodynamic changes.

Hyperglycaemia

Hyperglycaemia predisposes to diabetic microvascular disease, and treating hyperglycaemia can limit that progression and prevent disease development (as illustrated by the Diabetes Control and Complications Trial (DCCT) and the UK Prospective Diabetes Study (UKPDS).

Molecular consequences of hyperglycaemia

Advanced glycation end-products. Glucose and other glycated compounds can react with proteins and nucleic acids to give glycated products. The glycation occurs in a number of stages giving rise first to early reversible products and finally to advanced glycation end-products (AGEs). The long-term modification of proteins by non-enzymatic glycation and oxidation has been implicated in widespread pathology including macrovascular and microvascular disease (Fig. 1). AGEs modify the function of protein:

- intracellular proteins, by altering function
- extracellular matrix proteins, leading to abnormal interactions with other matrix elements and with matrix receptors
- plasma proteins, by causing binding to and activation of macrophages.

Tissue levels of AGEs increase with age, and they can also be derived from exogenous sources such as food and tobacco smoke.

Reactive oxygen species
Increased production of reactive oxygen species causes reduced availability of nitric oxide, with a loss of its anti-inflammatory, antiproliferative and anti-adhesive properties and an increase in proinflammatory factors (Fig. 1).

Activation of NFκB
NFκB is an intracellular transcription factor that mediates proinflammatory responses. Activation of NFκB can result from oxidative stress and from binding of AGEs to cell receptors on cells such as macrophages. This activation promotes vasoconstriction

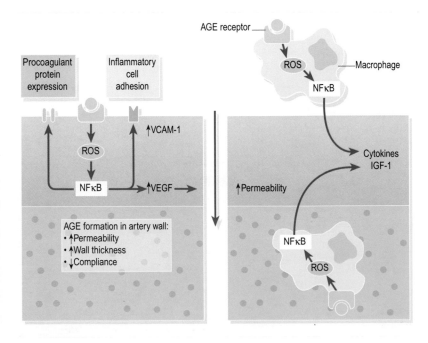

Fig. 1 **Schematic representation of impact of advanced glycation end-products on normal arterial cell wall homeostasis.** ROS, reactive oxygen species; AGE, advanced glycated end-products; NFκB, a transcription factor; IGF-1, insulin-like growth factor 1; VEGF, vascular endothelial growth factor; VPF, vascular permeability factor.

and expression of proinflammatory cytokines and procoagulants.

Sorbitol accumulation

Sorbitol is produced from glucose and NADPH through the action of aldose reductase (the polyol pathway). This reaction can have detrimental effects by reducing the availability of NADPH and by producing sorbitol inside cells. The latter can cause a fluid imbalance within the cells, potentially leading to disruption of cellular osmoregulation and cell function. The accumulation of the sorbitol in cells such as nerve or renal cells can damage the cells.

Activation of protein kinase Cβ

Intracellular glucose can lead to accumulation of diacylglycerol, which activates protein kinase Cβ in endothelial cells. This enzyme regulates vascular permeability, contractility and proliferation (Fig. 2). Its activation also causes release of vascular endothelial growth factor/vascular permeability factor, one of the possible prime culprits in diabetic eye disease.

Assessing average blood glucose levels with glycolated haemoglobin (HbA1c)

Glycosylation of haemoglobin (HbA1 or HbA1c) occurs as a non-enzymatic two-step reaction resulting in the formation of a covalent bond between the glucose molecule and the terminal valine of the β-chain of the haemoglobin molecule. The percentage of haemoglobin glycated is related to the prevailing glucose concentration. Glycated haemoglobin is expressed as a percentage of the normal haemoglobin (normal range approximately 4–8% depending on the technique of measurement). HbA1c provides an index of the average blood glucose concentration over the life of the

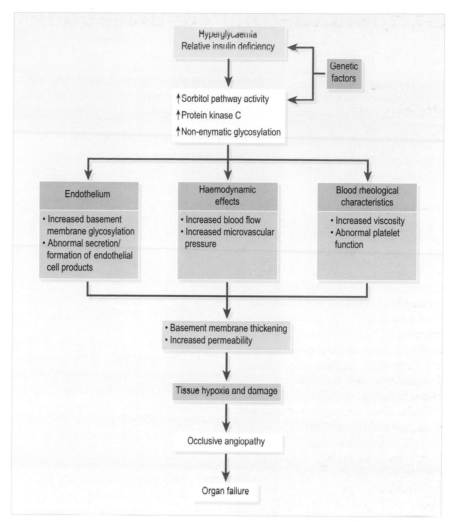

Fig. 3 **A possible pathogenic pathway of diabetic microangiopathy.**

haemoglobin molecule (a 6–12 week period) and so is an index of hyperglycaemia, and thus diabetes control, over that period. The figure will be misleading if the lifespan of the red cell is altered: altered red cell survival, as in renal failure, or an abnormal haemoglobin, as in thalassaemia. While HbA1c levels indicate if the patient's blood glucose levels, on average, are too high, they are not useful for day to day control; therefore, they should be used in conjunction with blood glucose monitoring. Glycated plasma proteins ('fructosamine') can also be measured as an index of control. Glycated albumin, the major component of glycated plasma proteins, and fructosamine levels relate to glycaemic control over the preceding 2–3 weeks. These assessments are useful in patients with a haemoglobinopathy, in pregnancy

(when haemoglobin turnover is changeable) and in situations that require rapid changes of treatment.

Haemodynamic changes

In diabetes mellitus, there are several changes to blood flow through vessels. There is an increased blood viscosity, increased shear stress, plugging of capillaries by activated leukocytes, closure of capillaries and proliferation of new vessels. This appears to result in a chronic hypoxia. These mechanisms are particularly illustrated in retinal disease (Fig. 3). New vessels grow in an attempt to bring blood back to the periphery of the retina. These vessels do not have the characteristics of the other retinal vessels and are inadequate at revascularizing ischaemic areas. They develop from the venous side of the retinal circulation, bleed easily and cause the growth of a reactive fibrous tissue.

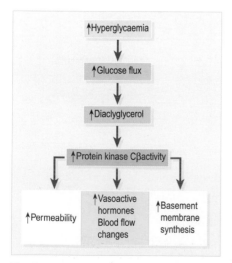

Fig. 2 **Impact on blood vessels of glucose-induced increase in protein kinase Cβ activity.**

Complications II: pathophysiology

- Hyperglycaemia alters intracellular and extracellular factors adversely.
- Hyperglycaemia activates intracellular sorbitol pathways, cell kinase and transcription factors.
- Hyperglycaemia alters extracellular haemodynamic and rheological properties.
- Protein glycation alters protein function.

Avoiding vascular complications

In industrialized countries, macrovascular disease is the major cause of mortality. Risk factors associated with a predisposition to macrovascular disease include diabetes mellitus and impaired glucose tolerance, hypertension, obesity, hypertriglyceridaemia and a decreased HDL cholesterol. The linkage of these factors is known as the metabolic syndrome (p. 64). For the practising physician, there are three implications in identifying the syndrome in any single patient:

- identification of any one of the changes should lead to a search for other features
- management of a diabetic patient should comprise management of blood glucose plus the other factors, such as hypertension and dyslipidaemia, that are important in predisposing to vascular consequences
- management of each patient with type 2 diabetes mellitus must be tailored to allow for the particular risk factor profile identified in that individual.

Thus, diabetes mellitus is no longer viewed as a disease of sugar alone; a more holistic approach is required if patients are to benefit from the information acquired through recent studies.

The major modifiable risk factors of macrovascular or microvascular disease in diabetes are:

- high blood glucose
- hypertension
- dyslipidaemia
- cigarette smoking.

The British study UKPDS found that improved control of blood glucose or blood pressure reduced the risk of:

- major diabetic eye disease by one quarter
- serious deterioration of vision by nearly one half
- early kidney damage by one third
- strokes by one third
- death from diabetes related causes by one third.

Control of blood glucose in prevention of vascular disease

Studies from Scandinavia, Japan, America (DCCT) and the UK (UKPDS) have identified intensive blood glucose control as an important factor in

limiting development and progression of diabetic microvascular and, to a lesser degree, macrovascular disease.

UKPDS

UKPDS involved more than 5000 patients with type 2 diabetes mellitus. Patients on intensive drug therapy had better blood glucose control than patients on conventional treatment irrespective of type of drug therapy or insulin, with a decreased risk of microvascular complications in the intensively treated type 2 diabetic patients (Fig. 1). The significant differences are shown in Table 1.

DCCT

DCCT demonstrated that intensive care aimed at optimal glycaemic control reduced the risk of developing microvascular complications (Figs 2 and 3) in type 1 diabetic patients. For example, the risk of developing retinopathy was reduced by 76% and the risk of progression of retinopathy by 50% in the intensively treated group. Intriguingly after the study, the difference in retinopathy risk remained significantly different at up to 4 years

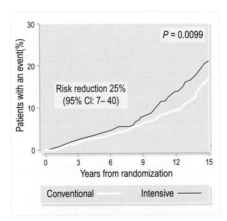

Fig. 1 **Development of microvascular complications.** Events were renal failure or death, vitreous haemorrhage, photocoagulation. (With permission from UKPDS.)

Table 1 **The effect of intensive therapy to control glucose in type 2 diabetes**	
Event	Risk reduction (%)
Any diabetes-related endpoint	12
Myocardial infarction	16
Retinopathy at 12 years follow-up	21
Cataract extraction	24
Microvascular endpoints	25
Albuminuria at 12 years follow-up	33
With permission from UKPDS.	

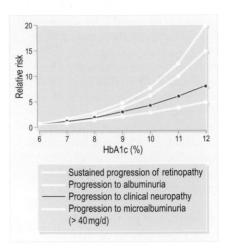

Fig. 2 **Microvascular complication are related to hyperglycaemia (as indicated by HbA1c).** (From Pickup J, Williams G 2003. Textbook of Diabetes Blackwell Publishing, with permission.)

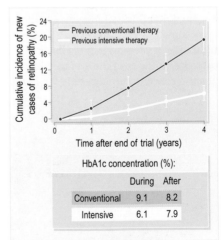

Fig. 3 **Microvascular complication are related to the duration of disease.** (From Pickup J, Williams G 2003. Textbook of Diabetes Blackwell Publishing, with permission.)

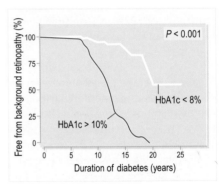

Fig. 4 **Hyperglycaemic memory.**

despite comparable blood glucose control (Fig. 4).

Summary

UKPDS in conjunction with DCCT and other studies confirmed the glucose hypothesis unequivocally. For every 1% fall in HbA1c there is a reduction in microvascular risk by about 25% irrespective of whether the patient has type 1 or type 2 diabetes mellitus. However, not all patients with optimal glycaemic therapy will be protected from complications. In neither DCCT nor UKPDS did intensive blood glucose control have an impact on macrovascular events.

Control of blood pressure

Treatment of hypertension in diabetics is based on the value of treatment in non-diabetic subjects studied in large randomized controlled studies. The UKPDS study showed that tight blood pressure control in patients with hypertension and type 2 diabetes mellitus achieved a clinically important reduction in the risk of deaths related to diabetes and incidence of microvascular complications (Table 2 and Fig. 5).

When the blood pressure is > 130 mmHg systolic or > 80 mmHg diastolic, the risk of complications of hypertension increases. So current proposals are to aim for these levels. In the MICRO-HOPE study, diabetic patients over the age of 55 years with one additional cardiovascular risk factor benefited from therapy with the angiotensin converting enzyme inhibitor ramipril. There was a 25% reduction in the combined risk of myocardial infarction, stroke and cardiovascular death.

Control of blood cholesterol

Plasma lipoprotein profiles in patients with type 2 diabetes mellitus tend to differ from healthy non-diabetic subjects

- ↑ large very low density lipoproteins (VLDL) type 1
- ↓ small VLDL-2

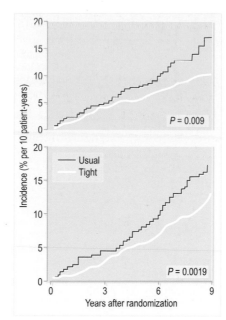

Fig. 5 **Treating hypertension.** Microvascular complications (top) and diabetes related death (bottom) according to tight or usual blood pressure control. (From Pickup J, Williams G 2003. Textbook of Diabetes Blackwell Publishing, with permission.)

- ↑ small low density lipoproteins (LDL)
- ↓ large LDL
- ↓ large HDL-2
- ↑ small HDL-3.

The extent of vascular disease in patients with type 2 diabetes mellitus is such that it may be reasonable to treat them in a similar way to those with established cardiovascular disease. In one study, even diabetic subjects without previous clinical heart disease had a similar risk of myocardial infarction as the non-diabetic subjects with previous myocardial infarction. There are substantial benefits in reducing mortality by reducing blood cholesterol levels using fibrates or statins:

- simvastin produced a 55% reduction in the incidence of major coronary

events in diabetic men with high LDL-cholesterol and previous coronary heart disease (mean follow-up 4.5 years)

- pravastatin over 5 years significantly reduced the incidence of coronary heart disease events in diabetic patients with average LDL-cholesterol and previous coronary disease.

The Heart Protection Study showed that even patients with diabetes and a 20% cardiovascular risk in the next 10 years can benefit from simvastatin despite having normal cholesterol (< 5.2 with LDL-cholesterol < 3.0 mmol/L).

Fibrates are an alternative to statins and may prove superior in selected cases since they reduce triglycerides and increase HDL.

Smoking

Smoking is one of the most potent risk factors for cardiovascular disease. Stopping smoking could reduce the risk of progression to cardiovascular disease by up to 70% in the non-diabetic population and we have no reason to believe that the benefit will be less in diabetic patients.

Use of aspirin in high-risk patients

Patients with a risk of cardiovascular events of > 20% in the next 10 years have a reduced mortality with aspirin, in the absence of contraindications. In the diabetic patient with angina, meta-analysis has confirmed that the benefits of aspirin therapy for secondary prevention are equivalent to those seen in non-diabetic patients. The benefit outweighing the risks of bleeding as a side-effect. For patients intolerant of aspirin, clopidogrel is a reasonable alternative, as shown in the subgroup analysis of the Clopidogrel in Unstable Angina to Prevent Recurrent Events (CURE) Trial.

Event	Risk reduction (%)
Any diabetes-related endpoint	24
Diabetes related deaths	32
Retinopathy progression	34
Microvascular disease	37
Stroke	44
Deterioration of vision	47
Heart failure	56
With permission from UKPDS.	

Table 2 **The effect of controlling blood pressure in type 2 diabetes**

Control of blood glucose

- Improving blood glucose control, by whatever means, decreases the risk of microvascular complications in type 2 diabetes without an adverse effect on macrovascular disease.
- Improving blood glucose control by intensive insulin therapy and education decreases the risk of microvascular complications in type 1 diabetes mellitus.
- Blood pressure control in patients with hypertension and type 2 diabetes mellitus reduces the risk of death and of diabetes-related complications.
- Statins and aspirin can be effective in reducing coronary events in diabetic patients.

Diabetic neuropathy

Hyperglycaemia is important in causing microvascular disease, but other risk factors such as hypertension (especially for renal and eye disease) and smoking (especially for renal disease) are also significant. Microvascular disease has a particular clinical impact through leading to neuropathy.

Diabetic neuropathy is the most common complication of diabetes mellitus. The main patterns of neuropathy are (Fig. 1):

- acute sensory nerve disorders: usually asymmetrical mononeuropathies and transient
- chronic sensory nerve disorders: usually symmetrical polyneuropathies
- acute motor neuropathies: uncommon
- autonomic neuropathy: most common clinical manifestation is erectile dysfunction.

The earliest functional change in diabetic nerves is delayed nerve conduction velocity. The earliest histological change is segmental demyelination, caused by damage to Schwann cells. In the early stages, axons are preserved, implying prospects of recovery; however, at a later stage, irreversible axonal degeneration develops.

Chronic sensory polyneuropathy

Chronic symmetrical sensory polyneuropathy is the most common form of diabetic neuropathy. Early clinical signs are loss of vibration sense, pain sensation (deep before superficial) and temperature sensation in the feet. At later stages, patients may complain of a feeling of 'walking on cotton wool' and can lose their balance when washing the face or walking in the dark owing to impaired proprioception. Involvement of the hands is much less common and results in a 'stocking and glove' sensory loss. Complications include unrecognized trauma at pressure points, beginning as blistering caused by an ill-fitting shoe or a hot water bottle, and leading to ulceration. Unbalanced traction by the long flexor muscles leads to a characteristic foot, with a high arch and clawed toes. This, in turn, leads to abnormal pressure distribution, resulting in callus formation under the first metatarsal head or on the tips of the toes and perforating neuropathic ulceration (Fig. 2). Neuropathic arthropathy (Charcot's joints) most often affects the ankle but may develop in any joint. It should be suspected in any neuropathic foot that becomes acutely swollen. Charcot's arthropathy is a severe complication with a high risk of eventual amputation as the foot structure becomes disorganized. Radiographs reveal disorganization of the bones, which once remodelled result in a deformed foot, for example with a rocker bottom deformity or a swollen disorganized knee (Fig. 3).

Acute sensory neuropathies

Acute sensory neuropathies may be (i) diffuse and painful or (ii) focal; in either event they are usually transient. A diffuse, painful neuropathy is uncommon. The patient describes burning or crawling pains in the feet, shins and anterior thighs, and muscular leg cramps. All symptoms are typically worse at night, and pressure from bedclothes may be intolerable (called **allodynia**). Painful neuropathy may present at diagnosis or develop after sudden improvement in glycaemic control. It usually resolves

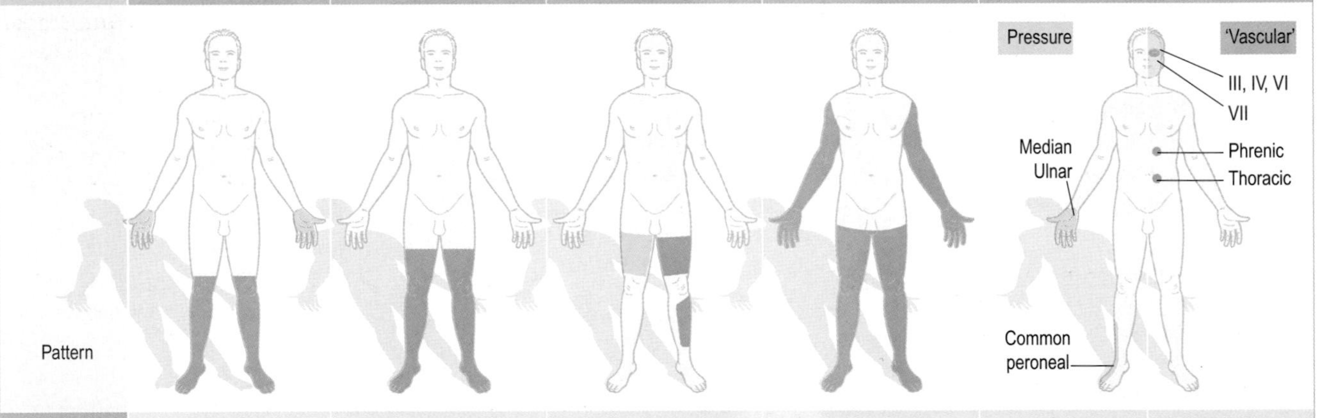

Syndrome	Chronic insidious sensory neuropathy	Acute painful neuropathy	Proximal motor myopathy	Diffuse motor neuropathy	Focal nerve palsies	
Pattern					Pressure Median Ulnar Common peroneal	'Vascular' III, IV, VI VII Phrenic Thoracic
Sensory loss	+ ➤ ++	+	0	0 ➤ +	++	++
Pain	0 ➤ +++	+++	+ ➤ +++	0	++	0 ➤ ++
Tendon reflexes	↓	↓	↓	↓	+	+
Muscle wasting and weakness	0 ➤ ++	+ ➤ +++	+++	++ ➤ +++	+ ➤ +++	0 ➤ ++
Autonomic features	+ ➤ ++	May be present	May be present	May be present	May be present	May be present
Prevalence and relationship to glycaemia	Common; usually unrelated to glycaemia	Relatively rare; onset often during hyper-glycaemia	Relatively rare; onset often during hyper-glycaemia	Relatively rare; generally unrelated to hyperglycaemia	Relatively rare; generally unrelated to hyperglycaemia	Relatively rare; sometimes related to hyperglycaemia

Fig. 1 **Clinical patterns of diabetic peripheral neuropathy.**

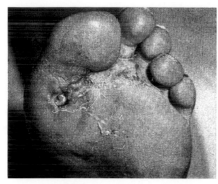

Fig. 2 **Neuropathic ulceration of the feet.**

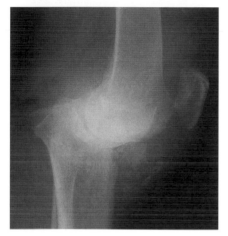

Fig. 3 **Radiograph of Charcot's arthropathy of the knee.**

spontaneously after 3 months and has resolved in 90% at 2 years. A more chronic form, developing later in the course of the disease, is sometimes resistant to almost all forms of therapy. There is no diagnostic test so alternative diagnoses such as vitamin B_{12} deficiency, alcohol, HIV-related, drug-related (isoniazid, nitrofurantoin), porphyria and cancer-related neuropathy should be considered. Muscle wasting is not a feature and objective signs can be minimal.

Focal *mononeuritis* and mononeuritis multiplex (multiple mononeuropathy) can affect any nerve in the body. Typically the onset is abrupt and sometimes painful. Radiculopathy (i.e. involvement of a spinal root) may occur. Isolated cranial nerve palsies to the external eye muscles, especially the third and sixth nerves, are more common in diabetes mellitus . A characteristic feature of diabetic III nerve lesions is that pupillary reflexes are often retained owing to sparing of pupillomotor fibres and the neuropathy may be painless. Full spontaneous recovery is the rule for most episodes of mononeuritis. Lesions are more likely to occur at common sites for external pressure palsies or nerve entrapment (e.g. the median nerve in the carpal tunnel). The carpal tunnel syndrome is a common cause for sensory symptoms in the hands in diabetes mellitus.

Acute motor neuropathies

Diabetic amyotrophy, is a motor neuropathy that is rare and more prevalent in older men. Presentation is with weight loss, painful wasting, usually asymmetrical, of the quadriceps muscles and depression. Depression may be severe and resolves as the weight increases. The wasting may be very marked and knee reflexes are diminished or absent. The affected area is often extremely tender. Extensor plantar responses sometimes develop and cerebrospinal fluid protein content is elevated. Diabetic amyotrophy is usually associated with periods of poor glycaemic control and may be present at diagnosis. It resolves like an acute sensory neuropathy with the same management regimen. Non-diabetic causes for the amyotrophy must be excluded including spinal lesions.

Autonomic neuropathy

Asymptomatic autonomic changes can be demonstrated on laboratory testing in many patients, but symptomatic autonomic neuropathy is rare. It affects both the sympathetic and parasympathetic nervous system and can be disabling. Patients with a severe autonomic neuropathy have an increased mortality possibly caused by cardiorespiratory arrest and more likely in those with marked prolongation of the QTc interval on ECG.

Cardiovascular system. Vagal neuropathy results in tachycardia at rest and loss of sinus arrhythmia.

Cardiovascular reflexes including the Valsalva manoeuvre are impaired. Postural hypotension results from loss of sympathetic tone to peripheral arterioles. Peripheral vasodilatation leads to a warm foot with bounding pulses.

Gastrointestinal tract. Vagal neuropathy can cause gastroparesis, often asymptomatic but rarely resulting in intractable vomiting. Diarrhoea often occurs at night with urgency and incontinence. Bacterial overgrowth in the stagnant bowel can lead to diarrhoea and steatorrhoea.

Bladder involvement. Vagal neuropathy can cause bladder stasis, loss of tone and incomplete emptying (predisposing to infection), with eventual urinary retention.

Erectile dysfunction. This is a common complication of diabetes mellitus, resulting from autonomic neuropathy, vascular disease or, more often, a combination of both. Acute illness, for whatever reason, can lead to transient impotence. Sexual dysfunction is also a feature in women, though its management is not yet clearly determined. Incomplete erections are a common presentation in diabetes mellitus. Another symptom is absent emissions caused by retrograde ejaculation in patients with autonomic neuropathy. However, erectile dysfunction in diabetes mellitus has many causes, including anxiety, depression, alcohol excess, drugs, primary or secondary gonadal failure and hypothyroidism and is more common with age (Table 1). History and examination should focus on these possible causes.

Table 1 **Erectile dysfunction: psychogenic versus organic cause**

Suggests psychogenic cause	Suggests organic cause
Sudden onset, related to life event	Gradual onset
Specific situations (intermittent)	All circumstances
Normal nocturnal and early morning erections	Altered or reduced nocturnal and morning erections
Relationship problems	Normal libido and ejaculation (unless dysfunction caused by hypogonadism)
Problems during sexual development	Normal sexual development

Diabetic neuropathy

- Diabetes-related neuropathies may be acute or chronic.
- Acute neuropathies are often painful, asymmetrical and invariably transient.
- Chronic neuropathies are usually painless, symmetrical and chronic.
- Autonomic neuropathy is unusual but can have widespread effects.
- Erectile dysfunction is a common and treatable problem in diabetes.

Principles of examination

Clinical examination of a patient with diabetes mellitus follows a 'rule of three':

- focus on three aspects of secondary causes of diabetes mellitus: (i) endocrine disease (thyroid, adrenal or pituitary disease), (ii) liver disease, (iii) rare syndromes associated with diabetes and altered clinical phenotype
- focus on three aspects of diabetes: (i) risk factors for complications, (ii) complication of diabetes, (iii) complications of therapy
- focus on three aspects of risk factors for complications: (i) blood pressure, (ii) lipid deposits, (iii) body mass index
- focus on three aspects of risk factors for macrovascular complications: (i) cerebrovascular disease, (ii) cardiovascular disease, (iii) peripheral vascular disease
- focus on three aspects of risk factors for microvascular complications: (i) retinopathy, (ii) nephropathy, (iii) neuropathy
- focus on three aspects of therapy complications: (i) lipohypertrophy from insulin injections, (ii) liver and renal disease caused by therapy, (iii) myositis from statin therapy.

Annual examination

All diabetes patients should be reviewed, at least once per year, by a hospital clinic, a diabetes centre (often attached to a hospital), their general practitioner (GP) or a combination of these three. It is important for diabetes patients to have access to advice outside the routine clinic. The purpose of a diabetes clinic is:

- patient education
- optimize targets of therapy (e.g. blood pressure and blood glucose)
- screen for diabetes complications
- treat established complications.

Monitoring targets of therapy are:

- weight (body mass index (kg/m^2)
- height (especially in children with centile charts)
- urine for ketones, albumin and possibly microalbuminuria
- HbA1c, blood glucose, lipid profile, creatinine
- blood pressure
- smoking

General examination

Consider appearance and the possibility of hormone or liver disease or rare clinical syndrome. Examine each area of the body (Fig. 1) particularly the feet (Table 1).

Routine laboratory investigations

Routine tests should include:

- HbA1c (measure of recent blood glucose levels)
- blood lipid profile

- serum creatinine
- urine proteinuria.

The following should also be considered:

- liver function tests
- free thyroxine and thyroid-stimulating hormone
- autoantibodies: thyroid, gliadin, endomysial, adrenal, gastroparietal
- diabetes-associated autoantibodies: glutamic acid decarboxylase or islet cell
- urine microalbuminuria.

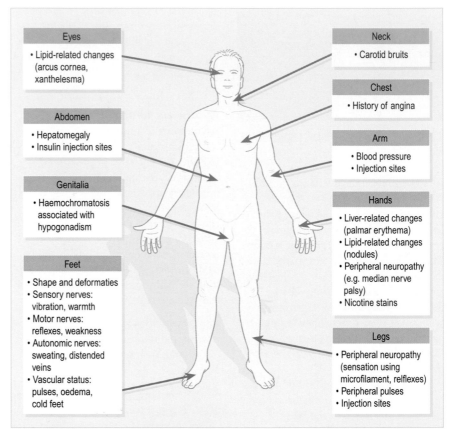

Fig. 1 **Examination of the diabetic patient.**

Area	Clinical examination	Objective testing
Shape and deformities	Toe deformities, prominent metatarsal heads, hallus valgus, Charcot deformity, callus	Radiograph of foot, foot pressure studies
Sensory function	Vibration (128 Hz fork), thermal proprioception, Semmes-Weinstein filaments	Biothesiometry, thermal-threshold testing
Motor function	Wasting, weakness, ankle reflexes	Electrophysiological tests
Autonomic function	Reduced sweating, callus, warm foot, distended dorsal foot veins	Quantitative sweat test, thermography for skin temperatures
Vascular status	Foot pulses, pallor, cold feet, oedema	Non-invasive Doppler and transcutaneous arterial oxygen studies

Table 1 **Examination of the foot in diabetic patients**

Examination for diabetic complications

Microvascular complications

Eyes

Visual acuity is always measured first. The pupils are then dilated with a mydriatic such as 0.5% tropicamide 30 minutes before ophthalmoscopy. Mydriatic drugs should not be used in patients with a history of glaucoma, except with the advice of an ophthalmologist. The ophthalmological examination begins at arm's length. At this distance, cataracts are silhouetted against the red reflex of the retina. The ophthalmoscope is advanced until the retina is in focus. The examination begins at the optic disc, moves through each quadrant in turn and ends with the macula (since this is least comfortable for the patient), requesting the patient to look into the light. The ophthalmoscope is then adjusted for examination of the cornea, anterior chamber and lens. Eye movements are also tested.

All patients with retinopathy should be examined regularly by a diabetologist or ophthalmologist. Early referral to an ophthalmologist is essential in the following circumstances:

- deteriorating visual acuity
- hard exudates encroaching on the macula
- preproliferative changes (cotton-wool spots or venous beading)
- new vessel formation.

Kidneys

Urine is examined for protein using a dipstick. Remember that trace positive is not positive if fresh urine is used. Microalbuminuria can be tested using a specific dipstick, or the microalbumin:creatinine ratio can be tested by laboratories on a spot urine sample. Serum creatinine should be analysed annually. Referral to renal specialist is advised once the serum creatinine has reached 150 μmol/L.

Feet

The feet should be inspected to identify anatomical distortions, pressure points, injuries and ulcers. Footwear should also be assessed. Peripheral pulses and the peripheral nervous system are assessed (Table 1). Early referrals to a chiropodist, even if there are no ulcers, is advisable since prevention is possible.

Erectile dysfunction

Ask if there are problems with obtaining an erection, early morning erections, penetration or ejaculation. There is no point in simply asking if the patient has sex as the response may not be informative.

Macrovascular complications

Ask about angina ('Do you get chest discomfort on climbing stairs?') but remember that cardiac pain is often atypical in patients with diabetes mellitus. Ask about erectile dysfunction. Check blood pressure, pulse rate and rhythm; listen for bruits in carotids and palpate all peripheral pulses. If in doubt, it is often prudent to perform resting electrocardiography (ECG) and to refer early to a cardiologist.

Skin and joints

The skin is often affected in the diabetic patient but the changes cannot be readily classified as microvascular or macrovascular. Skin lesions associated with diabetes include necrobiosis lipoidica diabeticorum (Fig. 2) and granuloma annulare (Fig. 3). The skin

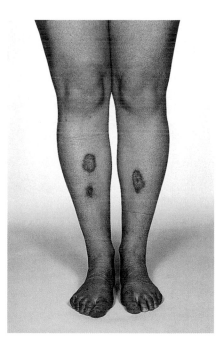

Fig. 2 **Necrobiosis lipoidica diabeticorum.**

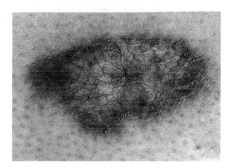

Fig. 3 **Granuloma annulare.**

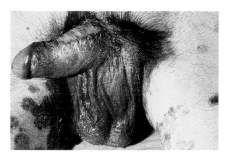

Fig. 4 **Features of the rash associated with a glucagonoma.**

may show lipohypertrophy or lipoatrophy caused by insulin injections. Other skin changes may be related to an underlying cause of secondary diabetes mellitus, such as 'bronze skin' caused by haemochromatosis or a rash associated with a glucagonoma (Fig. 4), Cushing's syndrome or acromegaly.

Thickening of the ligaments in the hands causes trigger finger or Dupuytren's contracture and is more common in diabetes mellitus. Thickened, waxy skin can be found on the backs of the fingers. These features may be caused by glycosylation of collagen and are not progressive. The condition is described as diabetic cheiroarthropathy. Joint contractures in the hands are also more common in patients who had childhood diabetes mellitus or who have poor diabetes control. The sign may be demonstrated by asking the patient to join the hands as if in prayer: the metacarpophalangeal and interphalangeal joints cannot be apposed.

> ### Principles of examination
>
> - Examination of a diabetic patient must be comprehensive.
> - Annual examination should focus on identification of complications and risk factors predisposing to microvascular and macrovascular disease.
> - Retinal examination requires skilled training, urine testing for nephropathy does not.

Management of neuropathy and infections

Diabetic neuropathies

Acute sensory neuropathies

Management must first exclude non-diabetic causes of neuropathy. Once diabetes mellitus is identified as the likely cause, four factors are important:

- reassurance about the high likelihood of remission within months
- management of blood glucose, with the introduction of insulin if control of glucose or pain is difficult
- reduction of the perception of neuritic pain: tricyclic antidepressants, gabapentin, and carbamazepine; topical capsaicin-containing creams help some patients; epidurals may be required for chronic unremitting pain
- multiple vitamins including vitamin B are used without clear evidence of their benefit.

Focal sensory mononeuropathies

Once again, reassurance about the high likelihood of remission within months is important. Management with insulin should be considered. Symptomatic treatments include eye patches for diplopia or wrist splints for carpal tunnel syndrome. Consider surgery for carpal tunnel syndrome and radiculopathy to decompress the lesions.

Acute motor neuropathies

The management of acute motor neuropathies is similar as that for acute mononeuropathies. General care including bed rest may be required when muscle wasting is severe.

Chronic sensory polyneuropathy

Management of at risk feet and foot ulcers is discussed on page 80. Charcot's arthropathy presents a particular problem. Management involves:

- immobilization
- custom-made footwear

- reconstruction (including realignment of unstable joints)
- intravenous bisphosphonates (which suppress osteoblast activity).

Autonomic neuropathy

Management varies with the system affected:

- *cardiovascular system:* debilitating hypotension can be helped by midodrine, fludrocortisone and erythropoetin
- *gastrointestinal tract:* bacterial overgrowth in the stagnant bowel can lead to diarrhoea and steatorrhoea; these symptoms can resolve dramatically with broad-spectrum antibiotics
- *bladder involvement:* urinary retention requires catheterization and infections should be treated aggressively with antibiotics.

Infections

Diabetic patients are more prone to a series of different infections including bacterial, fungal, urinary tract, skin and tuberculosis. Hyperglycaemia can affect the innate immune response, and this, allied to problems with blood supply and maintaining the skin surface structure, probably explains the excess risk for this broad range of infections. Equally, infections may lead to loss of glycaemic control and are a common cause of ketoacidosis. Insulin-treated patients need to increase their dose in the face of infection, and non-insulin-treated patients may need insulin therapy when they have an infection.

Infections occurring in diabetes mellitus include:

- staphylococcal infections (boils, abscesses, carbuncles)
- fungal infections (mouth, nails, skin folds)
- mucocutaneous candidiasis
- chronic peridontitis
- urinary tract infections
- pyelonephritis
- pneumococcal pneumonia
- tuberculosis.

Life-threatening infections in diabetic patients and their treatment are given in Table 1.

Table 1 **Life-threatening infections in diabetic patients**			
Type	**Causative factors**	**Treatment**	**Mortality (%)**
Malignant otitis external	*Pseudomonas aeruginosa*	Carbenicillin	10–20
Rhinocerebral mucormycosis	Fungi of the order Mucorales	Amphotericin B	34
Emphysematous cholecystitis	*Clostridia* sp. or *Escherichia coli*	Ampicillin/clindamycin	15
Emphysematous pyelonephritis	*E. coli* and others	Cephalosporins	10–37
Necrotizing fasciitis/cellulites	Mixed aerobic	Imipenem, debridement; hyperbaric oxygen	20
Non-clostridial gas gangrene	Mixed aerobic	Imipenem, debridement; hyperbaric oxygen	25–50

Management of neuropathy and infections

- Acute sensory neuropathies can be actively managed.
- Chronic sensory neuropathies are managed to limit structural damage.
- Certain symptoms of autonomic neuropathies can be treated.
- Certain infections are more common in diabetes.

Management of erectile dysfunction

All patients require counselling irrespective of the cause of the erectile dysfunction. Premature ejaculation and retrograde ejaculation should be managed by counselling. Vacuum devices provide a non-pharmacological aid for erectile dysfunction. A perspex tube with a seal in the base is placed over the penis and a vacuum pump draws blood into the penis to obtain tumescence. This is then maintained by slipping a rubber band over the base of the penis (then removing the tube) until intercourse is complete.

Drug therapy

Several classes of drug are available for erectile dysfunction.

Phosphodiesterase type 5 inhibitors

A therapeutic trial of phosphodiesterase type 5 inhibitors, including sildenafil (Viagra) or tadalafil, should be considered. These drugs enhance the effects of nitric oxide on smooth muscle and increase penile blood flow. They should be considered in most impotent diabetic patients who do not suffer from angina or previous myocardial infarction (concurrent use of nitrates is a contraindication). About 60% of patients will benefit (Fig. 1). Side-effects, including headaches and altered vision, are not uncommon.

Initial success could be followed by an attempt to achieve potency without the drug once self-confidence is restored. Since sometimes potency will continue unaided.

Prostaglandin E_1 preparations

Prostaglandin E_1 preparations also promote penile blood flow when applied topically to the urethra or as an intracavernosal injection. Alprostadil given, after suitable training, via a small pellet inserted into the urethra has a lower success rate than intracavernosal injection of the same drug but is less invasive. If the partner is pregnant, barrier contraception must be used to keep the prostaglandin away from the fetus. Patients can be trained to inject either alprostadil or papaverine (a smooth muscle relaxant), sometimes given

with phentolamine and moxisylyte (α-adrenoceptor blockers). The dose should be built up gradually until a satisfactory response is obtained. Side-effects include local reactions (e.g. discomfort, haematoma, fibrosis) and priapism. Patients should be given contact details for urgent treatment should erection last for more than 3 hours. To treat priapism, insert a large butterfly needle into the cavernous tissue and aspirate blood with a large syringe until detumescence has occurred.

Surgery

A proportion of patient find none of these therapies of value, especially if they have vascular disease. In which case surgery can be used to insert semi-rigid plastic rods into the penis so that penetration can be achieved (Fig. 2).

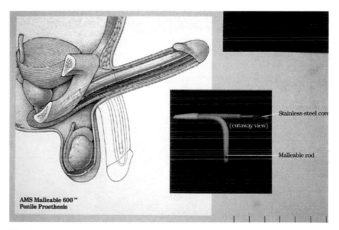

Fig. 2 **Plastic rod inserted surgically into the penis enables penetration if erectile dysfunction is unresponsive to other therapy. More sophisticated surgical devices are available including systems which can be manipulated to generate an erect penis when required.**

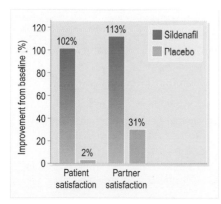

Management of erectile dysfunction

- All patients with erectile dysfunction need counselling.
- Premature ejaculation and retrograde ejaculation can be managed by counselling.
- Phosphodiesterase inhibitors and prostaglandin E preparations can be valuable.
- Vacuum devices and plastic rods provide a non-pharmacological alternatives for treatment.

The diabetic foot

Diabetic foot problems are responsible for nearly 50% of all diabetes-related hospital admissions and 10–15% of diabetic patients will develop foot ulcers at some stage in their lives. Half of all lower limb amputations are performed on people with diabetes mellitus. The risk of amputations is increased 15-fold in diabetes mellitus. Three factors are responsible for diabetic foot disease

- peripheral neuropathy
- peripheral arterial disease
- infection secondary to trauma or ulceration.

Although these factors may coexist, it is important to distinguish between the ischaemic and the neuropathic foot (Table 1), since a neuropathic ulcer invariably heals while the same is not true of ischaemic ulcers (Fig. 1).

The foot is at risk in a diabetic patient with:

- neuropathy
- ischaemia
- anatomical abnormality (e.g. hallux valgus)
- amputation or previous ulcer
- impaired mobility (e.g. age, stroke, arthritis)
- poor foot care.

Management of the diabetic foot

A diabetic patient should be referred to a chiropody or foot clinic with:

- callus, corns or ingrowing toenails
- ulcer
- significant ischaemia
- anatomical abnormality
- amputation or previous ulcer
- Charcot's arthropathy (Box 1).

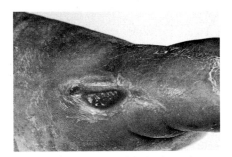

Fig. 1 **Ischaemic ulcer.**

Table 1 **Differential features of foot disease in diabetes mellitus**		
Features	Neuropathic foot	Ischaemic foot
Sensory defect	Yes	Not necessarily
Pulses	Present	Absent
Foot structure	Subluxed metatarsal heads (cocked toes)	Structure retained
Callus/ulceration	Excess callus formation at pressure points	Ulceration but not at pressure points
Plain radiograph	Plain radiograph may shows calcified arteries	

Box 1 *Charcot's Arthropathy*

Neuropathic arthropathy (Charcot's joints) may sometimes develop in any joint, but most often affects the ankle. It should be suspected in any neuropathic foot which becomes acutely swollen. Charcot's arthropathy is a severe complication with a high risk of amputation as the foot structure becomes disorganized. Radiographs reveal disorganization of the bones which results in a deformed foot such as a rocker bottom deformity, or a swollen disorganized knee. Treatment includes rest, immobilization, foot wear, constructive surgery (in expert hands) and possibly bisphosphonates.

Box 2 *Rules of foot care*

- Footwear must be carefully measured.
- Use lace-up shoes or trainers.
- Check before wearing for foreign objects.
- Wash feet daily and dry well especially between the toes.
- Cut nails carefully and regularly.
- Inspect feet daily especially on the soles.
- Use moisturizing creams for callus or fissures.
- Use chiropodist when appropriate.

Since diabetic foot problems are, by and large, preventable, the principles of foot care are important (Box 2). The four main threats to skin and subcutaneous tissues in the foot are:

- infection
- ischaemia
- abnormal pressure
- contamination.

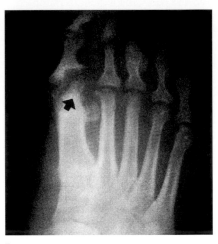

Fig. 2 **Radiograph with arrow pointing to area of osteomyelitis caused by infection in a diabetic neuropathic foot.**

They should be managed by a team to include a physician, a chiropodist and a vascular surgeon.

Infection

Infection must be treated early and aggressively. *Streptococcus pyogenes*, *Staphylococcus aureus* and anaerobic species are prevalent. Therapy includes:

- ulcer debridement
- callus removal
- protection of pressure points
- antibiotics.

Antibiotics must be broad based, moderately high dosage and given for prolonged periods, often in excess of 1 month, until infection is resolved. For deep or chronic infections, a radiograph of the feet should be taken to exclude osteomyelitis (Fig. 2).

Box 3 *Radiograph inflamed foot*

Radiograph inflamed or infected foot and search for gas from clostridial infection or evidence of osteomyelitis of bone.

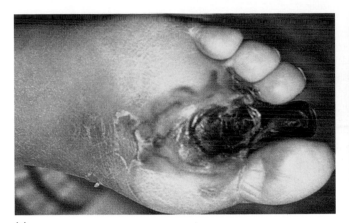

(a)

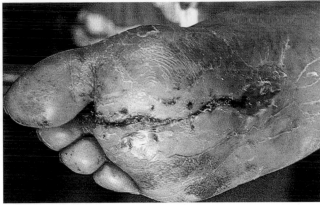

(b)

Fig. 3 **Necrotic toe.** (a) Before amputation; (b) after amputation using ray excision.

Table 2 **Antibiotics used in infected foot ulcers**	
Penicillin–cloxacillin combination	In view of the preponderance of staphylococci and streptococci in infected foot ulcers, either a penicillin–cloxacillin combination or alternatively, a cephalosporin (e.g. cefotaxime, cefuroxime) or a parenteral quinolone (e.g. ofloxacin) would be appropriate. Fusidic acid would be suitable as additional anti-staphylococcal therapy because of its particularly good tissue (including bone) penetration
Metronidazole	Evidence suggesting an anaerobic infection would necessitate the use of metronidazole. In the USA, clindamycin might well be given as a suitable alternative with the added benefit of activity against some aerobes.
Cephalosporin	Aerobic Gram-negative bacteria, excluding *Pseudomonas aeruginosa*, are likely to be sensitive to cefotaxime and cefuroxime (or a similar cephalosporin) and/or to an aminoglycoside or a parenteral quinolone.
Vancomycin	Vancomycin may be necessary for penicillin-resistant streptococci. Ciprofloxacin and oflaxacin have good activity against most aerobic pathogens but not against anaerobes, and imipenem has broad-spectrum activity which includes anaerobes.
Parenteral therapy	In more serious infections, and when surgery is necessary, inpatient management is obligatory, and antibiotics will be administered parenterally. However, in less severe cases, when there is no evidence of bone involvement and the patient is compliant, oral antibiotic therapy can be given on an outpatient basis.

and cultured dermis, the latter is like a skin graft but constructed from neonatal fibroblasts embedded in a synthetic matrix.

Amputation

Amputations are a last resort. They can be local (Fig. 3), involving a ray excision of the second, third or fourth toe and its associated metatarsal, or more radical, including above or below knee amputations of the limb. Considerable effort is required to walk with a prosthesis and this may be too much for the elderly, who are then confined to a wheelchair. In addition, the shift in weight can promote ulceration in the contralateral limb.

Osteomyelitis can be treated with long-term antibiotics but may require excision of the infected bone.

Ischaemia

The blood flow to the feet is assessed clinically, with Doppler ultrasound or, when severe and surgery is contemplated, by femoral arteriography. Arterial calcification will give false Doppler readings suggesting high blood flow. Localized areas of occlusion as shown on arteriography may be amenable to bypass surgery, stents or angioplasty; amputation is the last resort.

Abnormal pressure

Appropriate foot care, removal of calluses, rest and keeping any ulcerated site non-weight bearing are essential. A chiropodist can advise on the first two, which are aided by using moisturizing cream. Deep shoes and insoles can be especially constructed to help to move pressure away from critical sites; 'air-boots' or casts of the foot are also available. Weight bearing should be recommenced gradually, preferably with specially crafted foot wear or, as a less-satisfactory alternative, with sports trainers.

Wound environment

Dressings are used either to absorb exudate or to maintain moisture; in addition, they protect the wound from contamination. New techniques to promote healing of chronic ulceration are available. They are expensive and their role is to be established. They include platelet-derived growth factors

---

The diabetic foot

- Diabetic foot disease is caused by peripheral neuropathy and arterial disease and by infection secondary to trauma or ulceration.

- Anatomical abnormality or poor foot wear can lead to calluses and ulceration.

- Infections must be treated early and aggressively.

- Amputations are a last resort.

Diabetic eye disease

Patients with diabetes mellitus are at risk of eye disease including:

- *Diabetic retinopathy.* About 5% of patients in the past became blind after 30 years of diabetes, and diabetes mellitus is the commonest cause of blindness in the population up to 65 years of age.
- *Cataracts.* The lens may be affected by reversible osmotic changes in patients with acute hyperglycaemia, causing blurred vision. Senile cataracts develop 10 years earlier in diabetic patients compared with non-diabetic subjects. The risk can be reduced by improving blood glucose control.
- *Glaucoma.* Glaucoma is more prevalent in diabetes because of the new vessel formation in the iris (rubeosis iridis).
- *Ocular nerve palsies.* External ocular palsies, especially of the VI nerve, can occur. Like other causes of mononeuritis, these palsies are acute and transient, always resolving within 2 years and usually within 4 months.

The natural history of retinopathy

After 20 years of type 1 diabetes mellitus, almost all patients have retinopathy, while 60% progress to sight-threatening proliferative retinopathy. In type 2 diabetes mellitus, 20% of newly diagnosed patients already have diabetic retinopathy, and most will subsequently develop the condition. Without treatment, 50% of patients with proliferative retinopathy become blind within 5 years.

Diabetic retinopathy can be categorized as:

- background retinopathy
- preproliferative retinopathy
- proliferative retinopathy
- advanced diabetic eye disease
- maculopathy.

These categories are not distinct and there are other ways of classifying diabetic eye disease. Details within each category are shown in Figure 1 and Figures 2–5 illustrate each type.

Background retinopathy

Diabetes mellitus causes increased thickness of the capillary basement membrane and increased permeability of the retinal capillaries. Aneurysmal dilatation may occur in some vessels while others become occluded. These changes are first detectable by fluorescein angiography: a fluorescent dye is injected into an arm vein and photographed in transit through the retinal vessels. Clinically, these early abnormalities are visible through the ophthalmoscope as dot 'haemorrhages', caused by capillary microaneurysms. Leakage of blood into the deeper layers of the retina produces 'blot' haemorrhages, while exudation of fluid rich in lipids and protein cause hard exudates. Hard exudates have a bright yellow-white colour with an irregular outline and a sharply defined margin.

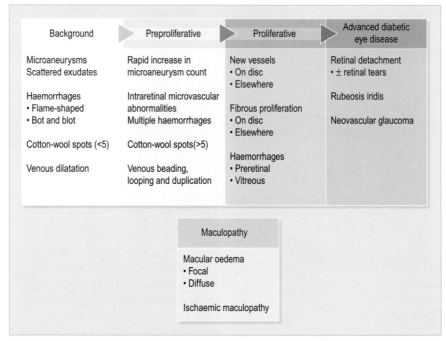

Background	Preproliferative	Proliferative	Advanced diabetic eye disease
Microaneurysms Scattered exudates	Rapid increase in microaneurysm count	New vessels • On disc • Elsewhere	Retinal detachment • ± retinal tears
Haemorrhages • Flame-shaped • Bot and blot	Intraretinal microvascular abnormalities Multiple haemorrhages	Fibrous proliferation • On disc • Elsewhere	Rubeosis iridis Neovascular glaucoma
Cotton-wool spots (<5)	Cotton-wool spots(>5)	Haemorrhages • Preretinal • Vitreous	
Venous dilatation	Venous beading, looping and duplication		

Maculopathy
Macular oedema • Focal • Diffuse
Ischaemic maculopathy

Fig. 1 **Stages of diabetic retinopathy.**

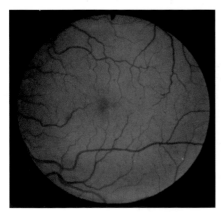

Fig. 2 **Mild background retinopathy.** (With the kind permission of Dr Massimo Porta.)

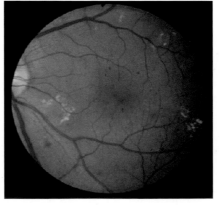

Fig. 3 **Moderate background retinopathy.** (With the kind permission of Dr Massimo Porta.)

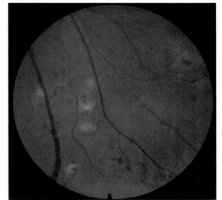

Fig. 4 **Proliferative retinopathy.** (With the kind permission of Dr Massimo Porta.)

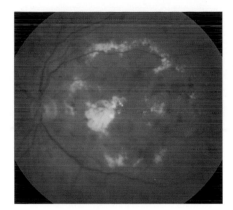

Fig. 5 Exudative maculopathy. (With the kind permission of Dr Massimo Porta.)

After 20 years of diabetes mellitus, virtually all fundi show at least the occasional microaneurysm on ophthalmoscopy. Background retinopathy does not in itself constitute a threat to vision but may progress to two other distinct forms of retinopathy: proliferative or maculopathy retinopathy. Both are the consequence of damage to retinal blood vessels causing retinal ischaemia.

Preproliferative retinopathy

Progressive retinal ischaemia can progress to preproliferative, sight-threatening retinopathy. The earliest sign is the appearance of 'cotton-wool spots', representing oedema resulting from retinal infarcts, also a feature of hypertensive retinopathy. Cotton-wool spots are grey–white, with indistinct margins, unlike hard exudates. Other changes include venous loops, beading, arterial sheathing and intraretinal microvascular abnormalities. These features are associated with a high risk of progression to proliferative retinopathy.

Proliferative retinopathy

New vessels are either superficial on the retina or grow forward into the vitreous. New vessels branch repeatedly, are fragile, bleed easily and may give rise to a fibrous tissue reaction. Haemorrhages can be preretinal or into the vitreous. A vitreous haemorrhage can cause loss of vision. Ophthalmoscopy shows a featureless, grey haze. Partial recovery of vision is the rule, as the blood is reabsorbed, but repeat bleeding may occur.

Fibrous proliferation associated with new vessel formation can distort the retina and the vision. Such changes may give rise to traction bands that contract, producing retinal detachment.

Table 1 **Management of retinopathy**	
	Management
Background retinopathy	Annual review by trained clinician or optician
Preproliferative retinopathy	Refer for specialist opinion
Diabetic maculopathy	Refer for specialist opinion
Proliferative retinopathy	Urgent specialist opinion
Diabetic maculopathy	Refer to specialist if there is an unexplained change in visual acuity or hard exudates within two disc diameters of visual fixation
Cataracts	Refer to specialist for cataract removal only when the patient finds the loss of vision interferes with their daily life

Diabetic maculopathy

Maculopathy mainly affects type 2 diabetic patients. There are three types of maculopathy:

- exudative
- oedematous
- ischaemic.

Of these, oedematous may be difficult to visualize with direct ophthalmoscopy and ischaemic is the least responsive to laser therapy. Macular oedema is the first feature of maculopathy and may in itself result in permanent macular damage if not treated early. Deteriorating visual acuity reveals the presence of significant retinopathy and may identify changes not seen on ophthalmoscope. It is essential to screen patients with diabetes mellitus regularly for changes in visual acuity.

Cataracts

Cataracts result in reduced visual acuity that cannot be improved by viewing through a pin-hole. Myotonic dystrophy and steroid therapy, which are associated with increased risk of diabetes mellitus, are also associated with cataracts. Juvenile or 'snowflake' cataracts are rare, diffuse, rapidly progressive cataracts associated with very poorly controlled diabetes mellitus.

Management of diabetic eye disease

Management of diabetic eye disease involves a close liaison between the medical team and the ophthalmologist (Table 1). Medical treatment to limit diabetic eye disease development or progression involves aggressive treatment of blood glucose and blood pressure levels. There is currently no specific medical treatment for background retinopathy. Smoking worsens the rate of retinopathy progression. Some evidence suggests that angiotensin-converting enzyme (ACE) inhibitors are of particular value in hypertension and the threshold for introduction of these agents should be low. Development or progression of retinopathy may be accelerated by rapid improvement in glycaemic control, pregnancy and in those with nephropathy; these groups need frequent monitoring.

Early referral to an ophthalmologist is essential in the following circumstances:

- deteriorating visual acuity
- hard exudates encroaching on the macula
- preproliferative changes (cotton-wool spots or venous beading)
- new vessel formation.

The ophthalmologist may perform fluorescein angiography to define the extent of the problem. Maculopathy and proliferative retinopathy are often treatable by retinal laser photo-coagulation; in the latter condition, early effective therapy reduces the risk of visual loss by about 50%. Treatment of disc new vessels is particularly successful using panretinal photo-coagulation. Surgery can be performed to try to salvage vision after vitreous haemorrhage and to treat traction retinal detachment in advanced retinopathy. Cataract surgery is highly successful but care must be exercised in the presence of active retinopathy given the risk of deterioration of the retinopathy, and laser therapy will be given concurrently in some instances.

Diabetic eye disease

- Almost all diabetes patients will progress to retinopathy over the long term; 60% progress to sight-threatening proliferative retinopathy.
- Maculopathy mainly affects type 2 diabetic patients.
- Medical treatment to limit development or progression of eye disease involves aggressive treatment of blood glucose and blood pressure levels
- Early effective therapy reduces the risk of visual loss by about 50%.

The diabetic kidney

The kidney can be damaged by diabetes in three main ways:

- glomerular damage
- ischaemia resulting from hypertrophy of afferent and efferent arterioles
- ascending infection.

Clinical nephropathy usually appears between 15 to 25 years after diagnosis and rarely develops 30 years from diagnosis. Nephropathy affects 25–35% of patients diagnosed with diabetes under the age of 30 years and is the main cause of renal failure in Europe, accounting for more than 30% of new renal replacement therapy. Some races such as African-Americans and South Asians are at particular risk of diabetic nephropathy. Patients with type 2 diabetes mellitus develop nephropathy less frequently than those with type 1 diabetes mellitus. Both proteinuria and diabetic nephropathy are associated with an increased risk of developing macrovascular disease. There is a strong genetic effect predisposing to nephropathy.

Natural history

The progression of diabetic nephropathy towards end-stage renal failure proceeds through five stages and does not become symptomatic until renal dysfunction is severe.

Stage 1: functional changes occur. Glomerular filtration rate and fraction are increased at diagnosis.

Stage 2: structural changes begin. Initially the glomerulus basement membrane is thickened. As the kidney is damaged, so the afferent arteriole (leading to the glomerulus) vasodilates more than the efferent glomerular arteriole. As a result, the intraglomerular filtration pressure increases, further damaging the glomerular capillaries. Increased intraglomerular pressure causes increased shearing forces and increased secretion of extracellular mesangial matrix material. This process leads to glomerular hypertrophy then sclerosis (Fig. 1).

Stage 3: marked by microalbuminuria. Disruption of the protein cross-linkages alters the glomerular filter, with progressive leak of large molecules into the urine. Small quantities of albumin

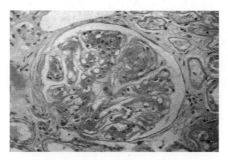

Fig. 1 **Glomerulus in diabetic nephropathy with pink staining tissue illustrating mesangial hyperplasia.**

can be detected in the urine and can be estimated on a 24-hour sample or, more practically, as an albumin:creatinine ratio from the first-voided urine sample (Box 1). Microalbuminuria may be tested for by radioimmunoassay or by using sensitive dipsticks; it is a predictive marker of progression to nephropathy in type 1 diabetes mellitus and of increased cardiovascular risk in type 2 diabetes mellitus.

Stage 4: overt clinical nephropathy. As glomerular filtration falls so blood pressure and plasma

creatinine rise and proteinuria increases (but not usually to levels associated with the nephrotic syndrome). Light-microscopic changes of glomerulosclerosis become manifest; both diffuse and nodular; the latter is known as the Kimmelstiel–Wilson lesion.

Stage 5: end-stage renal failure. Patients with nephropathy typically show: (i) anaemia (normochromic normocytic), (ii) altered calcium metabolism (low calcium, high phosphate), (iii) dyslipidaemia, (iv) hypertension.

Diagnosis

Proteinuria is the hallmark of diabetic nephropathy (Fig. 2). The urine of all diabetic patients should be checked annually for the presence of protein.

> ### Box 1 Definition of microalbuminuria
>
> Urinary excretion over 24 hours: 30–300 mg
> Urine albumin: creatinine ratio:
> > 2.5 mg/mmol (men) and > 3.5 mg/mmol (women).

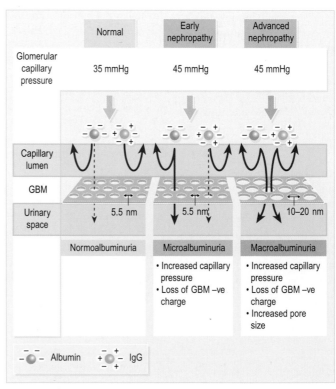

Fig. 2 **Evolution of proteinuria in diabetes.** Rising glomerular pressure leads to loss of the negative charge on the glomerular basement membrane (GBM) and increases in pore sizes; this allows passage of plasma proteins such as albumin and IgG, which are normally restricted.

Many centres also screen younger patients for microalbuminuria, particularly within 30 years of diagnosis, since good glycaemic control, early antihypertensive treatment and the use of an ACE inhibitor at this stage may delay progression to renal failure. Since there is no diagnostic test for diabetic nephropathy, including renal biopsy, other possible causes should be considered. Renal biopsy might be required, but in practice it is rarely necessary or helpful. Investigations to detect other causes of nephropathy

Tests for non-diabetic causes of nephropathy should also be carried out:

- urine microscopy for casts, red cells and culture
- serum protein electrophoresis
- serum calcium, phosphate, alkaline phosphatase, urate
- serum for autoantibodies including antinuclear factor
- renal ultrasound.

Infections
Urinary tract infections are more common in diabetes mellitus. Infections develop because of urinary stasis resulting from autonomic neuropathy affecting bladder function. Untreated infections in diabetic patients can lead to renal papillary necrosis, a rare condition in which renal papillae are shed in the urine and renal function deteriorates.

Management
The management of diabetic nephropathy is similar to that of renal failure from other causes. Particular attention must be paid to macrovascular risk factors and complications as well as the increased risk of neuropathy and retinopathy in patients with diabetic renal disease.

Blood glucose
Therapy should aim to achieve an HbA1c of < 7.0%. Once the creatinine has risen to 150 µmol/L, metformin should not be used, while the dose of other agents should be monitored carefully. Once the creatinine is > 200 µmol/L, only insulin therapy should be used.

Blood pressure
Aggressive treatment of blood pressure (target 130/80 mmHg) reduces the rate of deterioration to renal failure. ACE inhibitors are the drugs of choice at all stages including normotensive patients

with persistent microalbuminuria. Angiotensin II receptor blockers have a role when there is intolerance to ACE inhibitors. Combining an ACE inhibitor with a angiotensin-II receptor antagonist may provide superior blood pressure control. Loop diuretics are used in preference to thiazides once nephropathy is established. Combination therapy is usually required to achieve the blood pressure target.

Other therapy
Lipids. Once proteinuria is established, the risk of macrovascular disease is sufficient to warrant use of statins. The risk of myositis is increased in renal impairment when ciclosporin is used with statins or fibrates.

Smoking. Smoking predisposes to diabetic nephropathy and should be particularly avoided once nephropathy is established because of the risk of macrovascular disease.

Protein restriction. A reduction in protein dietary content to 0.7 g/kg daily is recommended but controversial.

General therapy
Once renal dysfunction has been established, therapy should include:

- phosphate binders such as calcium carbonate
- vitamin D analogues once serum parathyroid hormone increases
- erythropoietin once haemoglobin falls significantly
- multivitamins
- antacids such as ranitidine.

End-stage disease
Management of end-stage disease is made more difficult by the fact that patients often have other complications of diabetes mellitus such as blindness,

autonomic neuropathy or peripheral vascular disease. Once creatinine rises to > 500 µmol/L, renal replacement should be considered especially if symptoms develop. Plotting the inverse of creatinine against time gives an indication as to the rate of progression of renal dysfunction so that renal replacement can be planned in advance. There are three forms of renal replacement:

- continuous ambulatory peritoneal dialysis (CAPD)
- haemodialysis
- transplantation.

The usual initial therapy is CAPD. It is inexpensive compared with other replacement therapies, and it also avoids fluctuations in intravascular volume, a problem seen in patients with cardiac disease or autonomic neuropathy. Vascular access is not required, which is an advantage as vascular shunts tend to calcify rapidly in diabetic patients. Haemodialysis requires vascular access and is more prone to induce hypotension. Necrosis of digits can be a particular problem. Renal transplant is the treatment of choice and is with a cadaveric or, less frequently, live-related donor. Both patient survival and graft survival are slightly reduced in patients with diabetes mellitus. Assessment of the patients to exclude life-limiting co-morbidity, including macrovascular disease, is vital before a transplant is performed. A segmental pancreatic graft is sometimes performed at the same time as a renal graft. Although pancreatic transplants have a limited viability, owing to progressive fibrosis within the graft, they may give the patient a year or so of freedom from insulin injections.

The diabetic kidney

- Proteinuria is the hallmark of diabetic nephropathy and is a marker of cardiovascular risk.
- Microalbuminuria is a predictive marker of progression to nephropathy in type 1 and of increased cardiovascular risk in type 2 diabetes.
- Management of renal failure is similar to that from other causes.
- Blood glucose and blood pressure should be carefully controlled.
- Management of end-stage disease is made more difficult by co-occurrence of other complications of diabetes mellitus and by the slightly poorer rate of survival of graft and patient following transplants.

Emergencies in diabetes mellitus

Emergencies are very common and are rapidly fatal unless appropriate treatment is given. An altered conscious level or coma is a frequent presentation.

Causes of coma in diabetes mellitus

- hypoglycaemia
- diabetic ketoacidosis
- hyperosmolar non-ketotic (HONK) hyperglycaemia
- lactic acidosis
- uraemia
- non-diabetic causes.

Ketoacidosis

Diabetic ketoacidosis is usually caused by:

- undiagnosed diabetes
- stopping insulin therapy
- intercurrent illness.

The majority of cases reaching hospital could have been prevented by earlier diagnosis. The main errors are poor communication, education or management. In approximately 25%, the patients reduced or omitted insulin because they were not eating owing to nausea or vomiting. In this situation, insulin needs to be increased not reduced. Insulin should never be stopped without medical advice.

Pathogenesis

Ketoacidosis results from uncontrolled catabolism associated with insulin deficiency. Insulin deficiency must be present since only a minimal amount of insulin is sufficient to inhibit hepatic ketogenesis. Insulin deficiency causes increased hepatic glucose production, reduced peripheral glucose uptake by tissues such as muscle, and increased lipolysis. The second important feature is fluid depletion, resulting from the osmotic diuresis accompanying hyperglycaemia. Blood glucose may be 10–20 mmol/L in some patients, particularly in children, but is usually > 20 mmol/L.

The rapid lipolysis leads to elevated circulating free fatty acids. An excess of counter-regulatory hormone exacerbates the insulin deficiency and the two together lead to a series of reactions resulting in increased ketone bodies within hepatic mitochondria. This accumulation leads to metabolic acidosis. The excess ketones are excreted in the urine but also appear in the breath, producing a distinctive smell similar to that of acetone. Respiratory compensation for the acidosis leads to hyperventilation, described as 'air hunger'. Vomiting exacerbates loss of fluid and electrolytes. Progressive dehydration impairs renal excretion of hydrogen ions and ketones, aggravating the acidosis. As the pH falls below 7.0 ($[H^+] > 100$ nmol/L), pH-dependent enzyme systems in many cells are less effective Untreated, severe ketoacidosis is invariably fatal.

Symptoms and signs

The clinical symptoms of ketoacidosis are:

- vomiting (70%)
- thirst (55%)
- polyuria (40%)
- weight loss (20%)
- abdominal pain (15%).

The clinical signs are:

- dehydration
- tachycardia
- hypotension
- warm, dry skin
- hyperventilation (Kussmaul breathing)
- acetone on breath
- confusion, coma.

Investigations

Investigations in ketoacidosis include:

- blood glucose, creatinine and electrolytes, ketones
- full blood count
- arterial blood gases including pH,
- urine dipstick analysis for ketones, pyuria, blood, protein
- bacteriology: culture from blood, urine and a swab from any infection
- ECG to detect peaked T waves (hyperkalaemia), flat T waves (hypokalaemia) or undetected arrhythmia or infarction
- chest radiograph to detect infection or cardiac failure
- computed tomography or magnetic resonance scan if cerebral oedema is suspected or cause of coma unclear
- abdominal ultrasound
- exclude causes of coma and impaired consciousness other than diabetic ketoacidosis: stroke, postictal, cerebral trauma, alcohol intoxication, drug overdose.

Management

The principles of management are as follows.

Replace the insulin deficiency. Soluble insulin (6–10 U/h) is given as an intravenous infusion or by hourly intramuscular injections. The subcutaneous route is avoided because subcutaneous blood flow is reduced in shocked patients and insulin action is slower.

Replace the fluid losses. Normal saline is used, assuming 5 litre deficiency. Be cautious when treating patients at risk of cardiovascular disease and cardiac or renal dysfunction.

Replace electrolyte losses. Potassium levels must be monitored both with blood tests and by electrocardiograph (ECG). Although there is a total body potassium deficit initially, potassium levels in the blood may be high so potassium replacement is not given until the serum potassium is known. Intravenous potassium supplements, 40 mmol/L, are started when the serum potassium is in the normal range. Do not wait for the serum potassium to fall below the normal range.

Restore the acid–base balance. Both fluid replacement and insulin therapy will usually restore acid–base imbalance. Bicarbonate is controversial and seldom necessary and is only considered if the pH is < 7.0 ($[H+] > 100$ nmol/L) and is best given as an isotonic (1.26%) solution.

Seek the underlying cause. Physical examination and urine tests may reveal a source of infection. Note that fever is unusual even when infection is present. Polymorpholeucocytosis is present even in the absence of infection. ECG should be done to exclude a silent myocardial infarction, which can present with ketoacidosis.

Problems of management

Coma. General principles apply such as investigation of the cause (diabetic or non related; see above). Pass a nasogastric tube to prevent aspiration pneumonia since poor gastric emptying caused by gastroparesis is common.

Cerebral oedema. This rare complication is most prevalent in children or young adults. The mortality is high.

Hypotension. Hypotension may lead to prerenal failure. Plasma expanders (or whole blood) are, therefore, given if the systolic blood pressure is < 80 mmHg. A central venous pressure line should be considered. A bladder catheter is inserted if no urine is produced within 2 hours, but routine catheterization is not necessary.

Hypothermia. Severe hypothermia with a core temperature < 33°C may occur and may be overlooked unless a rectal temperature is taken.

Late complications. These include aspiration pneumonia and deep-vein thrombosis; they occur especially in the comatose or elderly patient. Anticoagulation therapy should be considered.

Complications of therapy. Hypoglycaemia and hypokalaemia can occur; excess fluid replacement causing cardiac dysfunction.

Subsequent management

Once blood glucose falls to 10 mmol/L, intravenous dextrose and insulin (3 U/h) are started until the patient can eat. At this stage, regular injections of subcutaneous insulin can be started. The intravenous infusion is then stopped and a similar amount of insulin is given as three injections of soluble insulin subcutaneously at meal times and a dose of intermediate-acting insulin at night.

Sliding-scale regimens usually reflect lack of familiarity with insulin dosage and may delay the establishment of stable blood glucose levels. Finally, the cause of the ketoacidosis should be confirmed with a review of the history and investigations and the patient advised how to avoid its recurrence.

Hyperglycaemic non-ketotic hyperosmolar states

Severe hyperglycaemia may develop without significant ketosis. These patients have type 2 diabetes mellitus so are usually adults and often with previously undiagnosed diabetes. Common precipitating factors causing HONK include drinking glucose-rich or 'energy' drinks, concurrent medication such as thiazide diuretics or steroids, and intercurrent illness. Non-ketotic coma and ketoacidosis represent two ends of a common spectrum, they are not two distinct disorders. The biochemical differences between the two conditions are caused by:

■ *age:* extreme dehydration characteristic of non-ketotic coma may be caused by less-severe thirst and more severe renal dysfunction in the elderly.

■ *insulin deficiency:* modest insulin deficiency found in type 2 diabetes means that endogenous insulin levels are sufficient to inhibit hepatic ketogenesis, while glucose production is enhanced.

Clinical features

Typically patients are adults with type 2 diabetes who present with severe dehydration and stupor or coma. Impairment of consciousness is related to the degree of hyperosmolality. As with diabetic ketoacidosis, an underlying illness must be sought. These patients are particularly prone to arterial thrombosis, leading to cerebrovascular accidents, myocardial infarction or arterial insufficiency in the lower limbs.

Treatment

Treatment is, with some exceptions, similar to that outlined for ketoacidosis. The differences are:

Osmolality adjustment. Because the plasma osmolality is usually extremely high, it must be estimated and monitored (normal range 275–300 mmol/kg).

Fluid replacement. Normal saline is the standard fluid for replacement. Avoid half-normal saline (0.45%) since rapid dilution of the blood may result in more severe cerebral damage.

Careful insulin use. Many patients are extremely sensitive to insulin and the glucose concentration may fall rapidly, resulting in cerebral oedema. If the glucose does fall, smaller dose of insulin (e.g. 3 U/h rather than 6 U/h) may be sufficient.

Anticoagulant prophylaxis. In view of the propensity of patients with HONK for arterial thrombosis, such therapy is particularly important.

Prognosis

Mortality in HONK may be as high as 20–30% in the elderly. Most patients, once they have recovered, can be managed with tablets and diet or even diet alone.

Emergencies in diabetes mellitus

Emergencies are very common and are rapidly fatal unless appropriate treatment is given.

Ketoacidosis

■ Ketoacidosis is associated with insulin deficiency.

■ Cardinal symptoms are polyuria, thirst, weight loss and weakness; drowsiness and coma follow.

■ Management comprises replacement of deficient insulin and of fluid and electrolyte losses.

Hyperglycaemic non-ketotic hyperosmolar states (HONK)

■ Adults present with severe dehydration and stupor or coma.

■ Treatment is similar to that outlined for ketoacidosis but osmolality, fluid and insulin levels must be monitored very carefully to avoid cerebral damage.

■ Patients with HONK are particularly prone to arterial thrombosis and so anticoagulant prophylaxis is advised.

Principles of management

Diabetes mellitus is the most common endocrine disease; over the long term, it causes tissue damage, seen clinically as complications. Effective care requires the patient to take responsibility for much of their own care and so good patient education and support are important. Management is focused on good risk factor control and detection of complications at an early stage. The broad approach includes education, diet, exercise, tablet therapy and, in selected cases insulin therapy.

Setting a treatment regimen

Ideal targets of therapy are given in Table 1.

Stepwise introduction of therapy

Diabetes therapy for hyperglycaemia is introduced in a stepwise manner; each further step is taken if the glucose fails to achieve the ideal HbA1c or fasting glucose target.

1. Diet and exercise
2. Diet, exercise and oral hypoglycaemic agent
3. Diet, exercise and combination of oral hypoglycaemic agents
4. Diet, exercise, combination of oral hypoglycaemic agents and insulin or
5. Diet, exercise and insulin.

Living with diabetes mellitus

Diabetic patients may have problems with specific aspects of daily life and the particular problems of a patient may influence the choice of treatment (Table 2). Issues related to specific at-risk groups, such as pregnant women, are discussed later in this section.

Work

All jobs are open to people with diabetes mellitus bar a few in which the risk of hypoglycaemia from insulin therapy might put others at risk (Table 3).

Finance

It is important that life and car insurance companies are informed of the diagnosis of diabetes mellitus on the start of insulin therapy. Some brokers are more interested in insuring such patients than others and will offer smaller premiums. The premium will be dependent on the type of insurance, the nature of the therapy, the risk of hypoglycaemia and the presence of complications. Visual acuity and fields must be assessed to determine suitability for driving. In the UK, patients with diabetes mellitus are exempt from prescription charges; their GP should sign a SP92 form to claim exemption. In the USA, patients may obtain cheaper medications from Canada (they can check websites).

Sport

People with diabetes mellitus can play and excel at most sports. Some sports are wary of allowing patients on insulin to participate in competition, such as scuba diving, motor rally and boxing. Patients exercising intensively are at risk of hypoglycaemia and should: (i) measure blood glucose before exercise; (ii) take 20 g carbohydrate every 45 minutes during exercise; (iii) keep fast-acting glucose preparations (such as Dextrosol in Europe) in their pocket for use if should they feel hypoglycaemic; (iv) avoid dangerous situations, such as swimming alone.

Holidays and travel

Patients with diabetes who are travelling will need:

- insulin, insulin syringes, glucose monitoring equipment; spare insulin and syringes when possible in case one is mislaid
- identification to confirm that they have diabetes (e.g. Medic Alert bracelet) and letter to confirm they can carry syringes in aeroplanes (such

Table 1 **Ideal targets of therapy**

Parameter	Recommendation
Weight: body mass index	< 25
Waist:hip ratio	
Men	< 0.95
Women	< 0.8
Glucose	
Fasting glucose	< 6.0 mmol/L (108 mg/dL)
Postprandial	< 6.7 mmol/L (120 mg/dL)
HbA1c	< 7.0%
Lipid profile[a]	
Cholesterol	< 4.8 mmol/L (185 mg/dL)
LDL cholesterol	3.0 mmol/L
Triglycerides	< 2.2 mmol/L (200 mg/dL)
Blood pressure	130/85 mmHg
Smoking	Nil

[a]Note that there is some variation in these targets between the American Diabetes Association and the European Diabetes Policy Group, e.g. the latter recommend a fasting triglycride < 1.7 mmol/L (150 mg/dL).

Table 2 **Some problems in the life of diabetic patients which may influence the choice of treatment**

Area	Examples
Employment	Shift-workers
	Long working day (early breakfast, late evening meal)
	Missed midday meal or frequent business lunches
	International travel
Eating	National variations (e.g. traditional large breakfast in UK, main meal at midday in some countries, dietary composition country to country, etc.)
	Individual variations (fads availability, affordability, preferences, eating out at restaurants)
Travel	Long-haul air travel
	Travel to work, e.g. long walk
Exercise	Sportsmen and women
	Sedentary office workers
	Labourers
Leisure	Strenuous hobbies, e.g. gardening, sport, etc.

Table 3 **Forms of employment from which insulin-treated diabetic people are generally excluded in the UK**

Employment	Examples
Vocational driving	Large goods vehicle (LGV), passenger-carrying vehicles (PCV), locomotives or underground trains, professional drivers (chauffeurs), taxi drivers (variable; depends on local authority)
Civil aviation	Commercial pilots, flight engineers, aircrew, air-traffic controllers
National and emergency services	Armed forces (army, navy, air force), police force, fire brigade or rescue services, merchant navy, prison and security services
Dangerous areas for work	Offshore oil-rig work, moving machinery, incinerator loading, hot-metal areas, work on railway tracks
Work at heights	Overhead linesmen, crane driving, scaffolding/high ladders or platforms

letters are not acceptable to the US Transportation Safety Authority, who require that labelled insulin vials or cartridges are carried together with needles)

- glucose tablets to avoid hypoglycaemia
- medical insurance.

Vaccinations should be done as required; there are no special needs when someone has diabetes.

On the day of travel for longer trips, patients should:

- aim to have a slightly higher blood glucose than usual; hypoglycaemia is very inconvenient
- check their blood glucose frequently
- be aware that the day is shorter if travelling eastwards; so the insulin dose may be too much and extra snacks may be required
- be aware that the day is longer if travelling westward; an additional insulin injection may be required, but only fast-acting soluble insulin should be used for the extra injection and blood glucose should be monitored carefully
- consider a change in regimen if the trip is very long, perhaps with stopovers, so that it is possible to use soluble insulin before each meal.

Driving
Patients with diabetes mellitus who drive a car or want to drive a car must:

- inform their car insurers as soon as they have been diagnosed; not to do so could invalidate any insurance
- check with other insurance brokers if the insurance premiums are increased following the diagnosis of diabetes
- inform the relevant licensing authority if being treated with tablets or insulin.

The UK DVLC will ask the patient to sign a declaration allowing their doctor to disclose medical information about them if they are treated with insulin. This point applies to motorcyclists and car drivers. Licences restricted to 1, 2 or 3 years are only provided if diabetes mellitus is treated with insulin.

To avoid hypoglycaemia, patients (particularly those taking insulin) should:

- be educated as to the nature and treatment of hypoglycaemia
- plan each journey and make provision for delays
- check their blood glucose before driving

- not drive for more than 2 hours; take regular breaks on long journeys and avoid fatigue
- should always carry glucose in the car
- have regular meals or snacks and not delay these
- if there are any suggestions that they are developing hypoglycaemic symptoms stop driving, switch off engine, remove ignition key and leave car
- always carry an identity card or bracelet
- never drink alcohol before driving.

Reasons for diabetic drivers to stop driving
Most people with diabetes obtain a license. Erratic diabetic control, hypoglycaemia and poor eye sight are the usual reasons for being refused a license. Patients with diabetes should not drive if they have:

- newly diagnosed diabetes, until glycaemic control and vision are safe
- just started insulin
- recurrent hypoglycaemia
- have impaired awareness of, erratic control of or difficulty with hypoglycaemic episodes
- have impaired vision not corrected with glasses
- have severe sensory peripheral neuropathy
- have severe peripheral vascular disease.

Surgery
Diabetic patients are at slightly greater risk of postoperative death as a result of their greater prevalence of heart disease. The control of blood sugar tends to be the focus of medical management after surgery, and the approach varies depending on the regimen the patient is using (Boxes 1 and 2). Control of blood glucose and electrolytes minimizes the risk of infection and balances the catabolic response to anaesthesia and surgery.

The general rules for surgery are:

- surgery is done by a team, liaison between the diabetes team and the anaesthetist is ideal

---

Box 1 Surgery diet- or tablet-treated diabetic patients

- Omit short-acting agents (e.g. sulphonylureas) on the morning of the operation.
- Omit long-acting sulphylureas (e.g. glibenclamide) 48 hours before the operation. Insulin may be required in place of them.
- Avoid glucose- and lactate-containing fluids in minor operations when possible.
- Avoid metformin perioperatively and if radiological contrast is required.
- For all major operations, consider need for insulin treatment.

Box 2 Surgery for insulin-treated diabetes

- Stop long- and/or intermediate-acting insulin the day before surgery; substitute short-acting insulin.
- Use intravenous 10% dextrose (500 mL infused at 100 mL/h) and soluble insulin (1–3 U/h) perioperatively with potassium chloride (10 mmol/L in 500 mL).
- Postoperatively, the infusion is maintained until the patient is able to eat. Other fluids must be given through a separate intravenous line.
- Glucose and potassium levels are monitored and the amounts in infusions are adjusted while keeping the infusion rate constant.

- metabolic control should be optimized before the operation; for emergency surgery, metabolic disturbances should be carefully managed
- hypoglycaemia should be avoided; insulin therapy is used when in doubt
- the patient is put at the beginning of the list at the start of the day
- electrolyte disturbances should be corrected before surgery, when feasible.

Principles of management

- Establish targets of therapy and work to achieve them.
- Educate patients to attain targets.
- Establish potential problems with work, finance, sport, holidays and driving.
- Educate patient about the problems associated with living with diabetes.

Non-pharmacological management

Although some patients may need drug or insulin therapy for effective control of their diabetes mellitus, some will achieve control on diet and exercise alone. However,

- diet and exercise are essential features of *all* diabetes regimens
- aerobic exercise improves insulin sensitivity
- aerobic exercise reduces cardiovascular risk.

Diet and lifestyle changes are the key to successful treatment of type 2 diabetes mellitus. If satisfactory metabolic control can be obtained by these means, then drug therapy may not be required.

Diet

The diet for a diabetic patient is, in principle, no different from the diet considered healthy for the population as a whole, except that refined sugar should be avoided. Particular attention should be paid to calories and the carbohydrate and fat content of the diet (Fig. 1).

Calories

Calories must be tailored to the individual but, in general, the total amount of calories should be provided in the diet as:

- 50–55% from carbohydrate
- 30–35% from fat
- 15% from protein.

Some recommend more carbohydrate and less fat. An overweight patient (BMI 25–30 kg/m^2) is started on a reducing diet of approximately 4–6 MJ (1000–1600 kcal) daily. A lean patient has an isocaloric diet. Reducing the energy content of a normal diet by 2100–4200 kJ will usually lead to a weight reduction of about 2 kg initially and of some 5–15 kg in total over the next 3 months. Patients who have lost weight because of untreated diabetes require energy supplementation.

Carbohydrate

Diets or food plans for diabetes should include unrefined carbohydrate rather than simple sugars such as sucrose. Carbohydrate is absorbed relatively slowly from fibre-rich foods, but blood glucose may rise rapidly when refined sugar is eaten. For example, the glucose peak seen in the blood after eating an apple is much flatter than that seen after drinking the same amount of carbohydrate as apple juice. The ratio of the area under the blood glucose curve after eating a particular food as a percentage of the area after taking the same amount of carbohydrate as glucose is termed the *glycaemic index*. Foods with a lower glycaemic index are preferable. For insulin-treated patients, estimating the carbohydrate content and glycaemic index of a meal can be valuable in estimating the insulin requirement.

Fats

The importance of cholesterol in the development of macrovascular disease has encouraged a more stringent attitude to fat content in diets than previously. However, low-fat diets, in general, have only a small impact on the serum cholesterol. Nevertheless, they can be of value in limiting increases in serum triglycerides. Saturated fatty acids should be restricted to less that 10% of the total daily energy intake. Foods that should be restricted but not eliminated include dairy produce, chocolate, ice creams, shellfish including prawns, the fat around meat, especially pork and lamb, fried foods, coconut oil, avocado and alcohol.

Prescribing a diet

Be sympathetic. Most people hate changing their diet. A diet history must be taken, and the diet prescribed should involve minimal interference with lifestyle. Patients taking insulin or oral agents should be advised to eat the same amount at the same time each day. Patients using insulin usually require snacks between meals and at bedtime, as injected insulin may linger in the blood. Alcohol is not forbidden, but its energy content should be taken into account; aim for < 28 units per week in men and < 21 units per week in women. Patients on insulin should be warned to

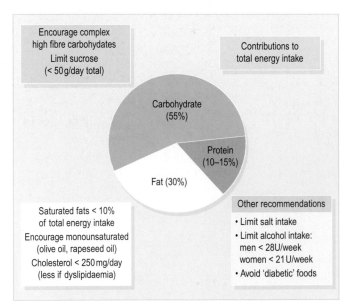

Fig. 1 **Dietary recommendations for patients with diabetes.**

Box 1 Diet

Artificial Sweeteners

Sweeteners are widely used and there is no evidence that they are deleterious. These non-nutritive sweeteners which are sugar-free are a valuable alternative to sugar to sweeten drinks and even to make cakes. They include aspartame, saccharin and acesulphame K.

Diabetic foods

Diabetic foods usually contain sorbitol or fructose to sweeten them. Large quantities can have side-effects such as diarrhoea, and they can cause appreciable glycaemia so they are not recommended.

Alcohol

As for the rest of us, alcohol can be drunk in moderation. Alcohol is a significant source of calories. In excess, alcohol can be dangerous as it can mask signs of hypoglycaemia.

Table 1 **Factors determining the glycaemic response to acute exercise in type 1 diabetes**	
Blood glucose	**Conditions**
Decreases	Hyperinsulinaemia exists during exercise
	Exercise is prolonged (>30–60 min) or intensive
	Less than 3 hours have elapsed since the preceding meal
	No extra snacks are taken before or during the exercise
	Generally remains unchanged
Exercise is brief	Plasma insulin concentration is normal
	Appropriate snacks are taken before and during exercise
Increases	Hypoinsulinaemia exists during exercise
	Exercise is strenuous
	Excessive carbohydrates are taken before or during exercise

avoid alcoholic binges since these may precipitate severe hypoglycaemia. A maximum daily salt intake of 2.3 g is recommended to limit the risk of hypertension. Diabetic foods are not recommended as they usually contain non-glucose refined sugars. Artificial sweeteners are useful and could be used as an alternative to sugar; concerns that they cause cancer have not been confirmed.

Exercise

Exercise, or rather lack of it, is a major cause of diabetes mellitus. It follows that exercise should be encouraged to limit the progression of diabetes. Certainly, exercise improves blood glucose control by improving insulin sensitivity; it can also reduce weight, blood pressure and dyslipidaemia. Most importantly, it can reduce the risk of cardiovascular disease. Exercise is, therefore, a cornerstone of diabetes therapy. The effect on blood glucose is described in Table 1.

When planning an exercise regimen it is important to:

- assess contraindications and limitations
- be realistic: people will only continue to do what they enjoy
- build up the amount of exercise gradually
- advise about the risk of hypoglycaemia
- remember any exercise is better than none.

Even the most simple advice can be of value, such as using the stairs, avoiding escalators and lifts, getting off the bus a stop early, walking faster, buying a dog.

Evidence from long-term lifestyle intervention trials suggests that lifestyle interventions are effective in the prevention of type 2 diabetes (see page 65). This was expected since lifestyle intervention focuses on the pathogenic mechanisms underlying the development of type 2 diabetes, in particular factors causing insulin resistance. Theoretically, it would be possible to prevent up to 70% of cases of type 2 diabetes in individuals at increased risk, if they could maintain normal body weight and engage in regular physical activity throughout their lives.

Box 2 gives guidelines for exercise in type 1 diabetes.

Box 2 Guidelines for exercise in type 1 diabetes

General advice
- Take exercise regularly; even walking has metabolic benefits.
- Tailor exercise to individual needs and physical fitness.
- Avoid hypoglycaemia during exercise by
  - taking 20–40 g extra carbohydrate before and hourly during exercise
  - avoid heavy exercise during peak from insulin injection
  - use non-exercising sites for injections
  - reduce pre-exercising insulin doses by 30–50% if necessary.

Cautions
- Take care if cardiovascular disease is also present.
- Those with peripheral neuropathy need to be aware of the potential for damage to the feet.

Contraindications
- In those taking insulin, sports where hypoglycaemia could be dangerous (e.g. diving, climbing, single-handed sailing, motor racing).
- Strenuous exercise in those with proliferative retinopathy (risk of possible haemorrhage).

Non-pharmacological management

Diet
- Diet should ideally contain no refined sugar and no diabetic foods.
- Small frequent meals are better.
- Calories, fat and salt intake should be limited.
- Alcohol use should be moderated.

Exercise
- Exercise improves blood glucose control by improving insulin sensitivity
- It can also reduce weight, blood pressure, dyslipidaemia and the risk of cardiovascular disease.

Pharmacological treatment I

Oral treatment for type 2 diabetes mellitus

Tablets are introduced when metabolic control cannot be obtained by diet and lifestyle changes alone. There are no strict rules regarding introduction of oral hypoglycaemic agents, the choice depends on individual patient's characteristics, the mechanisms of action of the available agents, therapy risk:benefit ratios and the degree of hyperglycaemia. Patients with baseline HbA1c 9% are less likely to achieve target HbA1c with monotherapy and are candidates for the early introduction of combination therapy. Patients not responding adequately to tablets will have been through the following stages: the drug of choice is used at low dose; the dose is increased; additional drugs are introduced in combination therapy to a maximum of two or three drugs; insulin is introduced usually in combination with metformin. The natural history of type 2 diabetes mellitus suggests that insulin secretory capacity is lost for up to 6 years after diagnosis and, therefore, the increase in blood glucose must be countered by a progressive change in tablet therapy.

Metformin

Metformin, a biguanide, is the drug of preference in the presence of obesity and insulin resistance. It reduces vascular risks in patients with diabetes mellitus. Metformin is associated with a 5–10% weight loss. The mechanism of action of metformin is unclear, but it decreases gluconeogenesis, and, hence, hepatic glucose output, and reduces fasting blood glucose (Fig. 1). Metformin may also increase insulin-stimulated glucose uptake in skeletal muscle. Metformin is an effective monotherapy for patients with elevated fasting blood levels. In patients with type 2 diabetes mellitus on insulin treatment, metformin can further reduce the HbA1c by approximately 1%.

Side-effects

The major side-effects are abdominal discomfort, nausea and diarrhoea; these problems are idiosyncratic but can be limited by initiating therapy gradually. Treatment should be started at a low dose of 250–500 mg per day and slowly increased to a dose of 500 mg three times a day. Hypoglycaemia is rarely a problem. Another rare complication of biguanides, of which metformin is a member, is the development of lactic acidosis, which is severe and potentially fatal. Metformin is, therefore, contraindicated in patients with renal or hepatic disease or where there is increased risk of lactic acidosis. In practice, metformin should not be used with a serum creatinine of >150 mmol/L. Metformin should be discontinued for 48 hours before and after radiological contrast use or surgical procedures. It should also be interrupted in severe illnesses.

Sulphonylureas

Sulphonylureas increase insulin secretion from the pancreatic beta cell by closing ATP-sensitive potassium (K_{ATP}) channels (Fig. 2), depolarizing the beta cell plasma membrane and increasing intracellular calcium concentration. It follows that sulphonylureas are of value when there is insulin secretory deficiency, but not when insulin resistance has a major impact. They are effective in decreasing both fasting blood glucose and postprandial hyperglycaemia (Fig. 3). Children with rare neonatal diabetes may have a mutation of the gene of KATP channels involved in insulin secretion and therefore respond to sulphonylureas. About 20% of patients have little or no glycaemic response to them and long-term failure rates are as high as 30%. *Tolbutamide* is the safest agent in the very elderly because of its short duration and weak action, though the tablet is large. *Glimepiride* is a more recently developed sulphonylurea with similar potency to other agents but the advantage of once daily administration, as has a long-acting formulation of *gliclazide*.

Important: be careful using sulphonylureas in the elderly.

Drug interactions and side-effects

Sulphonylureas bind to circulating albumin and may be displaced by other drugs that compete for their binding sites (e.g. warfarin). Side-effects can be either dose dependent or dose independent. Hypoglycaemia is the most common and dangerous side-effect in the former category, particularly during the late postprandial period or at night. Because many sulphonylureas persists for more than 24 hours, recurrent or

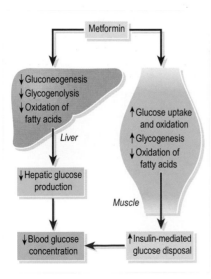

Fig. 1 **Mechanism of action of metformin.**

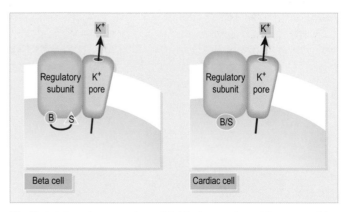

Fig. 2 **Sulphonylureas and meglitinides interaction with ATP-sensitive potassium channels.** S, sulphonylurea receptor; B, benzamido (e.g. meglitinides) receptor; cardiac cells have a receptor responding to both drug groups.

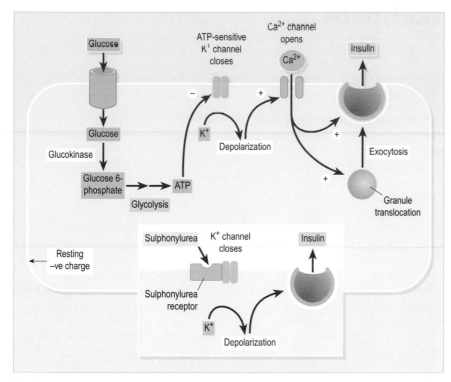

Fiɡ. 3 **Mechanism by which sulphonylureas and glucose stimulate insulin secretion.** GLUT, glucose transporter.

the beta cell membrane, increasing insulin secretion. Their action is more rapid in onset and less sustained than that of the sulphonylureas, so they can be taken shortly before each meal, significantly decreasing postprandial hyperglycaemia. The first of this class was *repaglinide*, which, because of its relatively short half life, has a limited effect on fasting glucose. Weight gain may be less than with sulphonylureas although full comparative studies with sulphonylureas are not yet available. *Nateglinide* is a novel agent derived from the amino acid D-phenylalanine. It acts directly on the pancreatic beta cells to stimulate rapid, glucose-dependent insulin secretion, which is rapidly reversed when glucose levels fall (Fig. 2). The effects of this class of drugs on mortality associated with macrovascular disease in diabetes mellitus is unknown.

Side-effects
There is a risk of hypoglycaemia during the late postprandial period with meglitinides.

prolonged hypoglycaemia is likely, and hospital admission is advisable. Of the dose-independent effects, skin rashes and weight gain are notable. Sulphonylureas should be used with care in patients with renal and liver disease, and only those primarily excreted by the liver (gliclazide) should be given to patients with renal impairment. Be careful with their use in the elderly, who are prone to serious hypoglycaemia. Avoid sulphonylureas once the creatinine rises to > 150 mmol/L.

Meglitinides
The meglitinides are a new class of compounds that can be used as initial monotherapy or in combination with metformin. Like sulphonylureas, they work by closing the K_{ATP} channels on

> ### Box 1
> UKPDS showed that improved blood glucose control, by whatever means (sulphonylurea, metformin or insulin), decreases the risk of microvascular complications in type 2 diabetes, without an adverse effect on macrovascular disease.

> ### Pharmacological treatment I
> - Metformin is the drug of preference in the presence of obesity and insulin resistance. It must be stopped 48 hours before and after radiological contrast use or surgical procedures.
> - Sulphonylureas are effective where there is insulin secretory deficiency rather than insulin resistance. They decrease both fasting blood glucose and postprandial hyperglycaemia. Not all patients respond to sulphonylureas, and they should be used with care in those with renal or liver disease and in the elderly, who are more susceptible to hypoglycaemia.
> - Meglitinides act similarly to the sulphonylureas, increasing insulin secretion but their action is more rapid in onset and less sustained. They can be taken shortly before each meal, significantly decreasing postprandial hyperglycaemia, but there is a risk of late postprandial hypoglycaemia. Meglitinides are valuable in patients allergic or sensitive to sulphonylureas.

Pharmacological treatment II

Diet and lifestyle changes are the key to successful treatment of type 2 diabetes mellitus. If satisfactory metabolic control can be obtained by these means then tablets may not be required. Tablets are introduced when metabolic control cannot be obtained by diet and lifestyle changes alone. There are no strict rules regarding introduction of oral hypoglycaemic agents, the choice depends on individual patient characteristics, the mechanisms of action of the available agents, therapy risk/ benefit ratios and the degree of hyperglycemia. The conventional tablet treatment in type 2 diabetes includes metformin and sulphonylureas. Recently new groups of drugs have been introduced. These include agents to promote insulin action (thiazolidinediones) and agents to inhibit food uptake (alpha-glucosidase inhibitors inhibits glucose uptake and orlistat inhibits fat uptake). The role of these agents in the treatment of impaired glucose tolerance remains unclear. Preliminary studies indicate that a thiazolidinedione or acarbose can limit the chance of progression to diabetes in patients with impaired glucose tolerance. Equally unclear is the role of these agents in diabetes. Since weight gain plays an important role in the progression to diabetes there is a case for using orlistat, which is used for lose weight, in the management of diabetes.

Thiazolidinediones (glitazones)

The thiazolidinediones (more conveniently known as the glitazones) act on the peroxisome proliferator-activated receptors (PPAR), particularly PPAR-γ. These nuclear receptors regulate DNA expression including genes involved in lipid metabolism (Fig. 1). The mechanism by which they increase insulin sensitivity in the peripheral tissues is unclear. Thiazolidinediones are effective in improving

Table 1	Guide to side-effect profile for any drug
Action	**Example**
Dose dependent	Hypoglycaemia with glucose-lowering drugs
Dose independent	Skin rashes can occur with most drugs
Drug entry point	Indigestion with metformin; local skin allergy for insulin
Drug metabolism point	Liver dysfunction with thiazolidinediones
Idiosyncratic	Cannot be guessed, such as weight gain with insulin, sulphonylureas and thiazolidinediones

glycaemic control in patients with insulin resistance and may be used as monotherapy or in combination with other antidiabetic agents (Table 2). Glitazones have a synergistic with metformin, showing that they act by a different mechanism. As monotherapy their glucose-lowering effect is similar to that of other oral agents, and they are used as monotherapy in the USA. In patients with type 2 diabetes mellitus on insulin treatment, glitazones can further reduce the HbA1c by about 1%, but care should be exercised because of fluid retention and this combination is not recommended in the UK.

Important: Be careful using thiazolidinediones with insulin therapy.

The thiazolidinediones are currently available for use as monotherapy or combined therapy in obese or non-obese subjects. However, in Europe metformin is currently the initial therapy of choice and thiazolidinediones are only used as monotherapy when metformin is not appropriate. Since thiazolidinediones improve insulin sensitivity and insulin secretion it follows that they can be used in conjunction with either metformin or a sulphonylurea. Whether thiazolidinediones can preserve insulin secretory function, as suggested by animal studies, remains unclear. The principles for starting therapy are similar to those employed for all these agents with a low dose being used initially, followed by a gradual increase in dose with careful monitoring for side-effects.

Particular care should be taken to check liver enzymes. Because thiazolidinediones require the presence of appreciable insulin to generate the glucose-lowering effect through enhanced insulin sensitivity it follows that they do not carry a high risk for inducing hypoglycaemia.

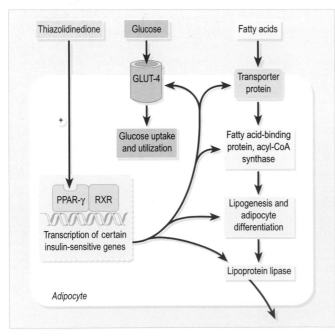

Fig. 1 **Mechanism of action of thiazolidinediones.** GLUT, glucose transporter; PPAR, proliferator-activated receptor; RXR, retinoid X receptor.

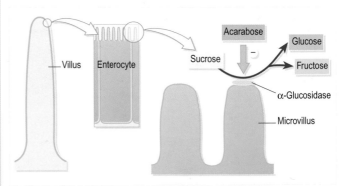

Fig. 2 **Action of α-glucosidase inhibitors (e.g. acarbose) at the intestinal brush border.**

Table 2 **Metabolic effects of thiazolidinediones**		
Muscle	**Adipose tissue**	**Liver**
Increased glucose uptake	Increased glucose uptake	Decreased gluconeogenesis
Increased glycolysis	Increased fatty acid uptake	Decreased glycogenolysis
Increased glucose oxidation	Increased lipogenesis	Increased lipogenesis

Thiazolidinediones can be used in mild renal dysfunction, in the elderly and in patients with polycystic ovary syndrome. They are contraindicated in pregnancy.

Side-effects

Troglitazone, the first thiazolidinedione to be used clinically, was associated with rare cases of hepatotoxicity and withdrawn. Regular liver function tests are, therefore, currently advised when using this group of drugs but the evidence suggests that there is not a group effect on liver function and the problem may have been unique to troglitazone. Thiazolidinediones can cause weight gain and fluid retention, even precipitating cardiac failure, particularly in patients on insulin therapy. Mild anaemia may also occur (Table 1).

Alpha-glucosidase inhibitors

Alpha-glucosidase inhibitors (e.g. *acarabose*) can reduce postprandial hyperglycaemia. They decrease the rate of digestion of complex carbohydrates in the small intestine (Fig. 2) and so they are generally ineffective in patients eating either very high or very low amounts of monosaccharides. The reduction in HbA1c levels is modest compared with other oral agents.

Alpha-glucosidase inhibitors can be used as monotherapy or in combination therapy with other anti-diabetic agents or with insulin. They have been used successfully to limit progression of impaired glucose tolerance and are particularly valuable when hyperglycaemia is mild and other agents might induce hypoglycaemia. Before starting treatment it is important to assess the potential benefit by confirming that the patient eats meals rich in complex carbohydrates. Subsequently, as with other diabetes therapy, the initial dose should be low and the drug titrated up slowly. The final dose is often limited by a patient's tolerance of gastrointestinal side-effects.

Side-effects

Undigested starch enters the large intestine where it is broken down by fermentation, causing abdominal discomfort, flatulence and diarrhoea. Dosage of α-glucosidase inhibitors (e.g. acarabose) needs careful adjustment to avoid these side-effects, which can severely restrict their clinical usefulness. As little or no acarbose enters the circulation (it is mainly inactivated in the gut) other side-effects are rare but liver dysfunction may rarely occur with high doses.

Anti-Obesity Drugs

Since the cause of type 2 diabetes is largely due to altered life-style the treatment should also be life-style related. Apart from diet and exercise, weight loss is desirable. Helping patients lose weight initially can be a valuable adjunct to the usual therapy. Many agents have been used to promote weight loss and two are currently on the market – orlistat and sibutramine.

Orlistat

Orlistat causes fat malabsorption by rendering intestinal lipase enzymes less effective; it, therefore, reduces the absorption of fat from the diet by about 30%. Orlistat can contribute to weight loss in patients who are already successfully maintaining a diet. Some of its benefit may be because it induces steatorrhoea in those who do not curtail their fat intake. Its place in diabetes management remains unclear.

In the Xendos trial, Orlistat successfully reduced the progression to type 2 diabetes in obese subjects with impaired glucose tolerance.

Side-effects

Steatorrhoea, even faecal incontinence, limits compliance with orlistat.

Sibutramine

Sibutramine enhances satiety. It does this by acting as a serotonin and noradrenaline reuptake inhibitor. Like Orlistat, Sibutramine enhances weight loss, and so should be used as an adjunct to diet and exercise. Sibutramine is not recommended as therapy to patients with uncontrolled hypertension.

Side-effects

Sibutramine is not addictive and has no known effect on heart valves as has been reported with other weight reducing agents. It may cause a small increase in blood pressure and pulse rate so it is not recommended in patients with hypertension which is not controlled.

> *Pharmacological treatment II*
>
> - Thiazolidinediones increase insulin sensitivity in the peripheral tissues and are effective in improving glycaemic control in patients with insulin resistance. They should be used cautiously in patients using insulin. They can cause weight gain and fluid retention, even precipitating cardiac failure.
>
> - Alpha-glucosidase inhibitors reduce postprandial hyperglycaemia by decreasing the rate of digestion of complex carbohydrates in the small intestine. They are of potential value in limiting progression from impaired glucose tolerance to diabetes.

Insulin treatment I

Insulin is found in every vertebrate. The active part of the molecule shows few species differences. Beef insulin differs from human insulin by three amino acid residues and readily induces antibody formation, whereas pork insulin, which differs by only one amino acid residue, is relatively non-immunogenic. Human insulin is rarely immunogenic. The aim of insulin therapy is to mimic insulin action in patients who have a relative or absolute insulin deficiency.

Indications for insulin treatment:

- type 1 diabetes mellitus
- type 2 diabetes mellitus when
  - tablets have failed
  - during illness
  - in acute myocardial infarction
- pregnancy when therapy other than diet alone is required.

Once insulin treatment is considered, several factors need deciding:

- type of insulin
- timing of injections
- dose of insulin
- education regarding adjustment of insulin dose
- need for assistance
- blood glucose monitoring
- education regarding hypoglycaemia
- need to carry glucose.

Insulin administration

Insulin is destroyed in the gastrointestinal tract and so must be given parenterally: usually subcutaneously but intravenously or intramuscularly in certain circumstances. One of the main problems is to avoid wide fluctuations plasma insulin and, thus, blood glucose. Insulin can be injected in several areas (Fig. 1). Injections should be rotated within the same region to avoid lipohypertrophy. Absorption is fastest from the abdomen (which is best suited to soluble insulin and rapidly acting

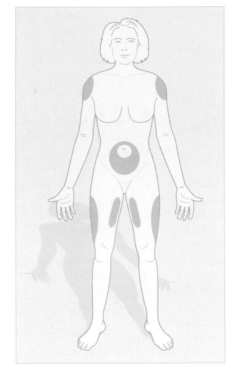

Fig. 1 **Insulin injection sites.**

forms) and slower from the thigh. The buttocks can also be used (particularly for long-acting insulin).

Errors in insulin injection technique

A number of problems can occur with injections:

- the wrong dose or timing
- air in the syringe
- poor injection technique
- injection into the wrong place (common), (e.g. into area of lipohypertrophy or an intradermal or intramuscular injection).

Types of insulin preparation

One of the main problems is to avoid wide fluctuations in plasma insulin and, thus, blood glucose. As a result, different formulations have been developed with differing onsets of action and action profiles (Table 1; Figs 2 and 3). The rate

of absorption of insulin from subcutaneous injection can be varied. Formulations available include:

- soluble rapid and short-lived effect
- rapid acting: analogues made to be absorbed and cleared rapidly
- prolonged acting: protein or zinc added to slow absorption
- slow release: analogues that precipitate at the pH of subcutaneous tissue to attempt to provide a supply closer to the physiological postprandial insulin release.

Soluble insulins

Animal insulins are still used widely in developing countries but have been now largely replaced in developed countries by biosynthetic human insulin. Human insulin is produced by adding a DNA sequence coding for proinsulin into cultured yeast or bacterial cells. Proinsulin is subsequently enzymatically cleaved to insulin. Soluble human or animal insulins have a similar pharmacodynamic profile, entering the circulation slowly, reaching a peak 60–90 minutes after injection and predisposing to hypoglycaemia several hours later as a result of persistent action. This profile differs from natural insulin which resembles monomeric insulin (see Fig. 2).

Rapid-acting insulin analogues

Insulin analogues have been manufactured in which the structure of the insulin molecule is modified to change its pharmacokinetics (Fig. 4).

Prolonged-acting insulins

Protein or zinc can be added to human and animal insulins to promote formation of insulin crystals. Crystals

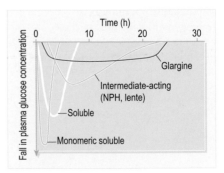

Fig. 2 **Action profiles of commonly used insulin preparations injected subcutaneously.** NPH, neutral protamine Hagedorn.

Table 1 **Characteristics of insulin preparations used in physiological insulin regimen**			
	Onset of action (min)	Peak of action (h)	Duration of action (h)
Mealtime insulins			
Soluble (regular)	≈ 30–60	≈ 2–3	≈ 6–8
Rapid-acting analogues (lispro, aspart)	≈ 20–30	≈ 1–2	≈ 3–4
Basal insulins			
Intermediate-acting insulin (e.g. NPH)	≈ 30–90	4–6	8–16
CSII (soluble or rapid-acting analogue)	≈ 20–60	Peakless	On demand
Insulin glargine	≈ 40–100	Peakless	16–24
CSII, continuous subcutaneous insulin infusion; NPH, neutral protamine Hagedorn.			

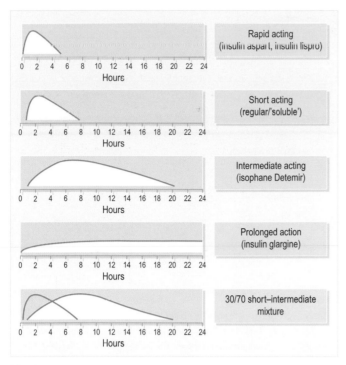

Fig. 3 **Approximate times and durations of action of various insulins following subcutaneous injection. Detemir has less of a peak in action than the isophane profile illustrated.**

dissolve slowly so these insulins appear cloudy. Protamine, isophane or NPH (neutral protamine Hagedorn) insulin, known as isophane insulin, can be premixed with soluble insulin to form stable mixtures. A range of these mixtures is available, but the combination of 30% soluble with 70% isophane is the most widely used.

Zinc insulins are prepared by precipitation of insulin crystals with excess zinc, thus delaying absorption and prolonging duration of action proportional to the size of the crystals. Since an excess of zinc is present in the vial, these insulins cannot be premixed with soluble insulin.

Insulin glargine has its structure modified to reduce its solubility at physiological pH, thus prolonging its duration of action (Fig. 4). It is injected as a slightly acidic (pH 4) solution and then precipitates in the tissues. The precipitates then dissolve slowly from the injection site, giving the preparation a longer duration of action and a less-peaked concentration profile in the blood than conventional long-acting insulins.

Other insulin delivery systems

There are a number of reasons continuous subcutaneous insulin infusion (CSII) pumps (Fig. 5) should be considered:

- poor metabolic control, with hyperglycaemia
    - poor metabolic control, with hypoglycaemia
    - instability of metabolic control, with swings from high to low glucose.

Alternative insulin delivery systems are at the experimental stage:

- transdermal insulin
- inhaled insulin
- buccal absorbed insulin
- intranasal insulin
- implantable insulin pumps to infuse insulin intravenously or intraperitoneally.

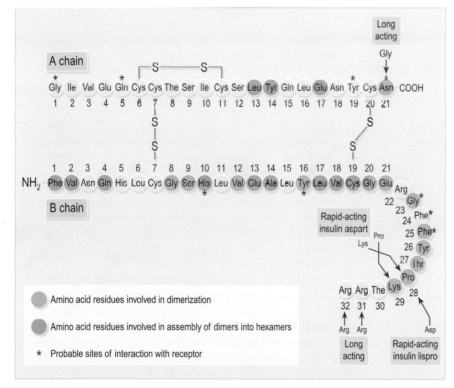

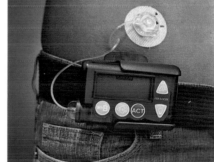

Fig. 4 **Modification to the primary structure of insulin in order to obtain rapid-acting (insulin lispro (Humalog) and insulin aspart (Novorapid)) or long-acting (insulin glargine) analogues.**

Fig. 5 **The insulin pump.**

Insulin treatment I

- Insulin therapy is not a cure for diabetes because it cannot mimic physiology.
- Insulin therapy is given using different regimens involving different injection frequency.
- Errors in injection technique are a common cause of deteriorating blood glucose control.
- Insulin analogues, pumps and new delivery systems reflect the problems with conventional insulin therapy.

Insulin treatment II

Insulin regimen and dose

Insulin regimen and dose must be individualized. There is no rule when it comes to the best regimen and the best dose. Some regimens are shown in Box 1.

Specific groups may require different therapy (e.g. young children (p. 104), the elderly (p. 106), in pregnancy (p. 102)). There is no evidence that multiple injections result in better HbA1c levels, but such regimens are more flexible and the risk of hypoglycaemia can be reduced.

Insulin regimens for type 2 diabetes

Adding insulin to tablet therapy may be required in patients with type 2 diabetes mellitus when glucose control is poor. Initially a small dose of intermediate acting insulin can be given, such as Insulatard insulin given at bedtime, in combination with oral hypoglycaemic drugs. This insulin inhibits hepatic glucose output overnight and can reduce HbA1c without an adverse effect on weight or hypoglycaemia risk. Long-acting insulin such as glargine can also be given as an alternative. Should bedtime insulin be insufficient, then a switch to regular twice daily insulin or more frequent injections, should be started, while maintaining metformin, which, on average, continues to have a beneficial effect.

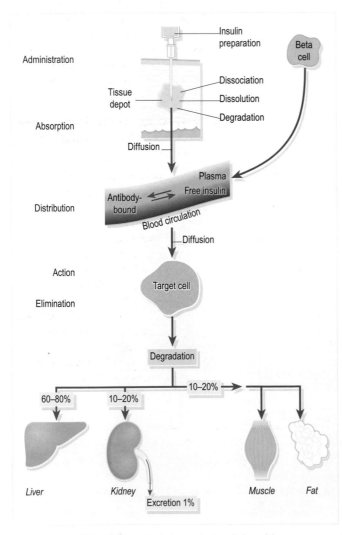

Fig. 1 **Processes affecting the availability of insulin.**

Box 1

Different regimes for insulin treatment include:

- Once daily injection with bedtime intermediate insulin for patients on diabetes tablets.
- Two times daily injections of fast-acting and intermediate-acting (or premixed) insulin.
- Three times daily injections including twice daily regimen plus midday fast-acting insulin.
- Four times daily injections including three times daily premeal fast-acting insulin and slower acting insulin (isophane, NPH, detemir or glargine) at bedtime.

Insulin availability

Many factors are known to affect insulin absorption, its availability to target tissues and its elimination (Fig. 1). Some factors can cause metabolic instability (Fig. 2):

- alterations in insulin pharmocokinetics (rare)
  - insulin antibodies binding insulin
  - insulin clearance over-rapid
- alterations in insulin action
  - insulin receptor defects
  - insulin postreceptor defects (e.g. obesity, type 2 diabetes)
- drugs
- counter-regulatory hormone disturbances.

Brittle diabetes mellitus

Brittle diabetes mellitus is used to describe patients with recurrent ketoacidosis and/or recurrent hypoglycaemic coma; however there is no precise definition. Most patients are those who experience recurrent severe hypoglycaemia. It was once said that there is no such thing as brittle diabetes only brittle diabetics. Certainly, once underlying causes and improvements in management have been implemented, attention should focus on psychosocial issues.

Recurrent severe hypoglycaemia

Each year, about 10% of patients taking insulin will have a severe hypoglycaemia requiring intervention by someone else. Approximately 1–3% of patients with type 1 diabetes mellitus have recurrent severe hypoglycaemia. Most patients with recurrent persistent problems are adults who have had diabetes mellitus for more than 10 years and have low production of endogenous insulin as estimated by C-peptide. Pancreatic alpha-cells are still present in undiminished numbers, but their glucagon response to hypoglycaemia is virtually absent and the catecholamine response may be impaired. These patients, therefore, lack a major component of the hormonal defence against hypoglycaemia (see Fig. 2). The following factors predispose to recurrent hypoglycaemia:

- over treatment with insulin
- frequent hypoglycaemia impairs the response to further hypoglycaemia within 2 weeks (Fig. 3)
- frequent hypoglycaemia lowers the blood glucose level at which symptoms develop

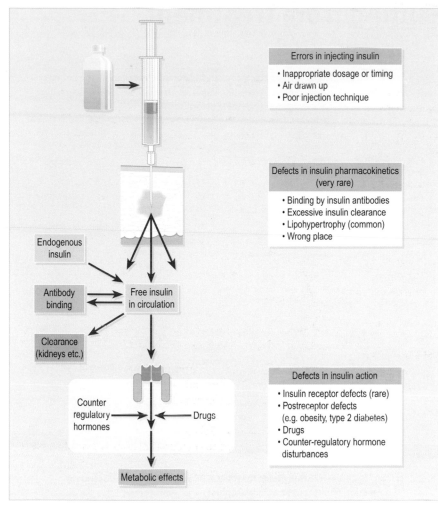

Fig. 2 **Possible causes of metabolic instability in insulin-treated patients.**

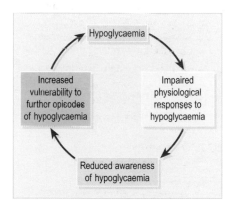

Fig. 3 **The vicious circle of repeated hypoglycaemia.**

- endocrine causes including pituitary insufficiency, adrenal insufficiency and premenstrual insulin sensitivity
- gastrointestinal causes including exocrine pancreatic failure and diabetic gastroparesis
- renal failure: the kidneys are important for the clearance of insulin and of oral hypoglycaemic drugs such as sulphonylureas
- patients: therapy can be manipulated or misunderstood.

Recurrent ketoacidosis

Recurrent ketoacidosis usually occurs in adolescents or young adults, particularly girls. Metabolic decompensation may develop very rapidly. A combination of chaotic food intake and insulin omission, whether consciously or unconsciously, is now regarded as the primary cause of this problem. It almost always occurs in the context of considerable psychosocial problems, particularly eating disorders. This area needs careful and sympathetic exploration in any patient with recurrent ketoacidosis. It is perhaps not surprising that, in an illness where much of one's life is spent thinking of and controlling food intake, 30% of

women with diabetes have had some features of an eating disorder at some time. Other causes include:

- *iatrogenic:* inappropriate insulin combinations may be a cause of swinging glycaemic control (e.g. a once-daily regimen may cause hypoglycaemia during the afternoon or evening and prebreakfast hyperglycaemia owing to insulin deficiency)
- *intercurrent illness:* unsuspected infections, including urinary tract infections and tuberculosis, may be present; thyrotoxicosis can also manifest as unstable glycaemic control.

Insulin dosage

Insulin dosage is largely idiosyncratic and there are only broad rules to apply. For treatment of ketoacidosis see page 84.

Intravenous soluble insulin can be given at a dose of 6 U/h (in children start at 0.1 U/h per kg body weight) during ketoacidosis; more may be required in the presence of infection, and less (about 0.5–1 U/h) once glucose control is established (see p. 86). Subcutaneous insulin is given as 0.5–1.5 U//kg daily in divided doses, initially trying the lower doses to limit the risk of hypoglycaemia. Doses over 2 U//kg dailyy almost always indicate an underlying problem.

Complications of insulin treatment

Complications of insulin treatment include:

- allergy (local or general): circulating insulin antibodies can affect insulin action
- dose-dependent effects
  - hypoglycaemia
  - weight gain (caused by the anabolic action of insulin)
- dose-independent effects
  - lipohypertrophy (caused by repeated injections at the same site)
  - lipoatrophy (rare now with purified insulin)
  - insulin oedema (especially with the introduction of insulin).

Hypoglycaemia resulting from treatment

Hypoglycaemia is the most common complication of insulin therapy and limits what can be achieved with insulin treatment. It is a major cause of anxiety for patients and relatives. Symptoms develop when the blood glucose level falls towards 3 mmol/L and typically develop over a few minutes, with most patients experiencing 'adrenergic' features of sweating, tremor and a pounding heart beat (Table 1; Fig. 1). Some physiological protection exists to limit the severity of hypoglycaemia (Fig. 2) but this response, particularly the release of glucagon and catecholamines, can be impaired in those who have had diabetes for a long time (over 10 years). These patients, therefore, lack a major component of the hormonal defence against hypoglycaemia.

Symptoms and signs

Physical signs include pallor and a cold sweat. Many patients with long-standing insulin-treated diabetes report loss of these warning symptoms and are at a greater risk of progressing to more severe hypoglycaemia. Such patients appear pale, drowsy or detached: signs that their relatives quickly learn to recognize. Behaviour is clumsy or inappropriate, and some become irritable or even aggressive. Others slip rapidly into hypoglycaemic coma. Occasionally, patients develop convulsions during hypoglycaemic coma, especially at night. It is important not to confuse this with idiopathic epilepsy, especially since patients with frequent hypoglycaemia often have abnormalities on the electroencephalogram. Another presentation is with a hemiparesis that resolves within a few minutes when glucose is administered. Hypoglycaemia is a common problem in patients on insulin treatment. Virtually all patients experience intermittent symptoms and one in three will go into a coma at some stage in their lives. A small minority suffer attacks that are so frequent and severe as to be virtually disabling. Hypoglycaemia results from an imbalance between injected insulin or inappropriate oral hypoglycaemic therapy and a patient's normal diet, activity and metabolic requirements. The times of greatest risk on insulin

Table 1	**Signs and symptoms of hypoglycaemia and actions to be taken by the patient**		
Symptoms	Physiological mechanism	Onset occurs at blood glucose (mmol/L)	Intervention required
Hunger, sweating, tremor, palpitations	Autonomic response to subnormal glycaemia	Below ~3.5	Take glucose-rich sweets, drink, or food
Cognitive dysfunction, incoordination, atypical behaviour, speech difficulty, drowsiness, dizziness	Neuroglycopenia (brain deprived of glucose)	Below ~2.8	Take glucose-rich sweets or drink, and seek assistance
Malaise, headache, nausea, reduced consciousness	Severe neuroglycopenia	Below ~2.0	Third party intervention required
Convulsions, coma	Severe neuroglycopenia	Below ~1.5	Medical intervention essential

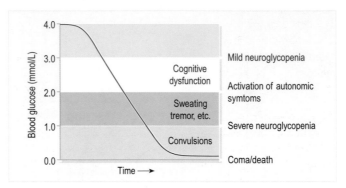

Fig. 1 **Glycaemic thresholds for release of adrenaline and subsequent activation of autonomic and neuroglycopenic symptoms.** As the glucose falls so more thresholds are passed and responses activated. In patients with hypoglycaemia unawareness, these threshold are reached at a lower glycaemic level if at all.

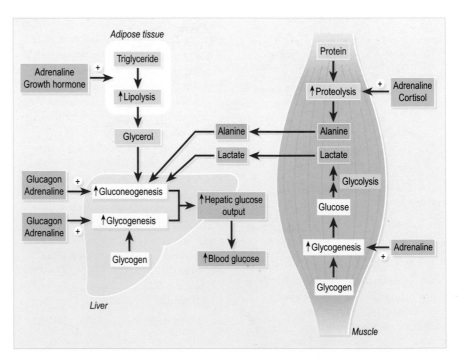

Fig. 2 **Metabolic action of counter-regulatory hormones in response to hypoglycaemia.** Of these hormones adrenaline is the most important, followed by glucagon and then growth hormone and cortisol. Adrenaline increases blood glucose by promoting lipolysis, gluconeogenesis, glycogenolysis (in liver and muscle) and proteolysis. Lipolysis and proteolysis promote liver gluconeogenesis.

are before meals, during the night and, for those taking sulphonylureas, during the late afternoon. Irregular eating habits, unusual exertion and alcohol excess may precipitate episodes; other instances in those on insulin therapy appear to result simply from variations in insulin absorption.

Hypoglycaemic unawareness

People with diabetes have an impaired ability to counter-regulate glucose levels after hypoglycaemia. The glucagon response is invariably deficient. The adrenaline response may also fail in patients with a long duration of diabetes, and this is associated with loss of warning symptoms. Recurrent hypoglycaemia may itself induce a state of hypoglycaemia unawareness; the ability to recognize the condition may sometimes be restored by relaxing control for a few weeks.

Nocturnal hypoglycaemia

Basal insulin requirements fall during the night but increase again from about 4 a.m. onwards, at a time when levels of injected insulin are falling. As a result, many patients awake with high blood glucose levels, but find that injecting more insulin at night increases the risk of hypoglycaemia in the early hours of the morning. The problem may be helped by:

■ checking that a bedtime snack is taken regularly
■ for patients taking twice daily mixed insulin to separate their evening dose and take the intermediate insulin at bedtime rather than before supper
■ reducing the dose of soluble insulin before supper, since the effects of this persist well into the night
■ changing patients on a multiple injection regimen with soluble insulin to a rapid-acting insulin analogue
■ using the new longer-acting insulin analogues with a flatter profile of action overnight may also prove of value.

Mild hypoglycaemia

Any form of rapidly absorbed carbohydrate will relieve the early symptoms, and sufferers should always carry glucose or sweets. Drowsy individuals will be able to take carbohydrate in liquid form (e.g. Lucozade). All patients and their close relatives need careful training about the risks of hypoglycaemia. They should be warned not to take more carbohydrate than necessary, since this causes a rebound to hyperglycaemia. The dangers of alcohol excess and hypoglycaemia while driving need to be emphasized.

Severe hypoglycaemia

The diagnosis of severe hypoglycaemia resulting in confusion or coma is simple and can usually be made on clinical grounds, backed by a bedside blood test. If real doubt exists, blood should be taken for glucose estimation before treatment is given. Patients should carry a card or wear a bracelet or necklace identifying themselves as diabetic, and these should be sought in unconscious patients.

Unconscious patients should be given either intramuscular glucagon (1 mg) or intravenous glucose (25–50 mL 50% dextrose solution) followed by a flush of normal saline to preserve the vein (since 50% dextrose scleroses veins). Glucagon acts by mobilizing hepatic glycogen and works almost as rapidly as glucose. It is simple to administer and can be given at home by relatives. It does not work after a prolonged fast. Oral glucose is given to replenish glycogen reserves once the patient revives.

Hypoglycaemia limits the intensity of blood glucose control using insulin. In the DCCT, those patients with good glucose control experienced increasing frequency of severe hypoglycaemia (Fig. 3). Therefore, diabetes control in patients receiving insulin is a compromise between risk of hypoglycaemia and risk of diabetes complications.

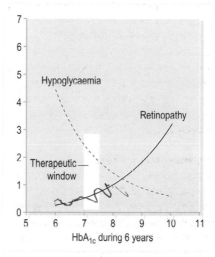

Fig. 3 **Risk of severe hypoglycaemia per year is higher with good glycaemic control (low HbA1c).** The DCCT showed that the risk of severe hypoglycaemia per year increased as the HbA1c fell. The therapeutic window is a theoretical target for HbA1c in patients that would balance the risks of hypoglycaemia and complications.

Hypoglycaemia resulting from treatment

■ Hypoglycaemia is the most common complication of insulin therapy; symptoms develop over a few minutes.

■ Patients and their families quickly learn to recognize and treat the symptoms of hypoglycaemia. Treatment depends on the severity of the hypoglycaemia.

■ In severe hypoglycaemia, the unconscious diabetic should be given either intramuscular glucagons or intravenous glucose.

■ Good glucose control lessens the chance of developing complications but is associated with an increasing frequency of severe hypoglycaemia.

Diabetes and pregnancy

Modern management of pregnancy in diabetic women means that pregnancy outcome in specialized centres approaches that in non-diabetic pregnancy. Yet in the 1960s, morbidity and mortality for both mother and child were substantial. This transformation has resulted from meticulous metabolic control throughout the three trimesters of pregnancy and general improvements in medical and obstetric management (Fig. 1).

Contraception and diabetes

Since pregnancy in diabetes should be planned, contraception is an important part of management. The options are as for non-diabetic individuals. The only point of relevance in diabetes relates to the metabolic side-effects associated with oestrogens, though these are minimal with low-oestrogen preparations. Therefore low-oestrogen preparations are preferable. However, in women with macrovascular disease or risk, combined oestrogen–progesterone contraception is avoided if possible.

Contraindications to pregnancy in diabetes

Contraindications include:

- clinical ischaemic heart disease
- advanced nephropathy
- active proliferative retinopathy
- severe symptomatic autonomic neuropathy.

Risks of diabetic pregnancy

Maternal risks include:

- metabolic deterioration
- microvascular complications can progress
- macrovascular complications
- risk of urinary tract infection increased
- risk of pre-eclampsia increased
- rates of Caesarian section increased.

Fetal risks include:

- risk of congenital malformations increased (cardiac, sacral agenesis, spina bifida)
- rates of stillbirth increased
- perinatal morbidity and mortality increased
- neonatal complications increased (fetal distress, jaundice, hypoglycaemia)
- risk of diabetes in later life increased.

Gestational diabetes

Gestational diabetes is a specific subcategory of diabetes mellitus when glucose intolerance develops during pregnancy and remits following delivery. There is no consensus as to the definition of gestational diabetes. It is classified as impaired glucose tolerance in pregnancy and incorporates undiagnosed pre-existing impaired glucose tolerance or diabetes. It is detected by the O'Sullivan screening test (Box 1). Table 1 shows two criteria used for diagnosing gestational diabetes mellitus.

About 2% of pregnant white Europeans develop gestational diabetes. Women are at particular risk if they have a previous history of gestational diabetes, are older or overweight, have a history of large-for-gestational age babies and belong to certain ethnic groups. Those with gestational diabetes are at high risk of subsequent gestational diabetes and progression to type 2 diabetes mellitus. A small percentage have diabetes-associated antibodies and progress to type 1 diabetes mellitus.

Gestational diabetes is usually asymptomatic. Treatment is with diet, though there are no data to support intervention other than possible reduction in the risk of macrosomia. About 30% of patients require insulin therapy during the pregnancy. Insulin does not cross the placenta. Oral agents such as metformin and second-generation sulphonylureas may be of value, though caution should be exercised and they remain the second line of choice. Gestational diabetes has been associated with the obstetric and neonatal problems described for pre-existing diabetes mellitus, with the sole exception that there is no increase in the rate of congenital abnormalities. The lack of congenital abnormalities in gestational diabetes is because of the later onset of glucose intolerance in that condition, consistent with these congenital abnormalities arising from glucose intolerance in the first trimester. Hospital admission is required if the patient is symptomatic, has ketonuria or a marked hyperglycaemia (>15 mmol/L).

Management of diabetes in pregnancy

When a pregnancy is planned, optimal metabolic control should be sought before conception to avoid congenital malformations (Table 2). Management will vary with the trimester (Table 3).

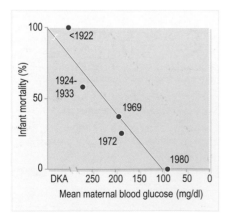

Fig. 1 **Correlation of mean maternal glucose concentrations and infant mortality found in published studies, 1922 to 1980.** As near-normal maternal blood glucose concentrations have been attained, infant mortality has decreased from 100% in the pre-insulin era to a rate close to that in nondiabetic pregnant women in the 1980s.

> ### Box 1 The O'Sullivan screening test
>
> Challenge with 50 g oral glucose
> Plasma glucose is ≥ 7.8 mmol/L at 60 minutes
> Sensitivity and specificity > 80% for glucose intolerance at 28 weeks.

Table 1 **Criteria for diagnosing gestational diabetes mellitus based on an oral glucose tolerance test**

	Plasma glucose (mmol/l)			
	Fasting	60 min	120 min	180 min
National Diabetes Advisory Board (1979)[a]	>5.8	>10.6	>9.2	>8.1
World Health Organization Criteria (1998)[b]	>7.0[c]	–	>7.8	–

[a]Based on a 100 g glucose test; positive diagnosis if two or more values raised.
[b]Based on a 75 g glucose test; positive diagnosis if 120 minute values is raised.
[c]Implies diabetes preceded the pregnancy.

The following eight points summarize the management strategy.

1. Prepregnancy counselling to optimize blood glucose control and thereby limit risk of congenital malformations.
2. Optimize blood glucose control with postprandial blood glucose between 4 and 7 mmol/L and HbA1c (or fructosamine) in the normal range.
3. Monitor blood glucose control. Ketoacidosis in pregnancy carries a 50% fetal mortality, but maternal hypoglycaemia is relatively well tolerated.
4. Dietary modification with limited calorie intake in obesity (30% decrease) and avoidance of refined carbohydrate.
5. Insulin therapy if blood glucose does not achieve targets. Do not use insulin analogues without counselling. Use multiple injections or insulin subcutaneous pump, as insulin requirement rises progressively during the second and third trimester.
6. Avoid oral hypoglycaemic agents unless strong indication.
7. Review in joint diabetes–antenatal clinic with diabetes physician and nurse plus obstetric team at intervals of 2 weeks or less. The aim should be outpatient management with a spontaneous vaginal delivery at term. Retinopathy and nephropathy may deteriorate during pregnancy. Expert fundoscopy and urine testing for protein should be undertaken at booking, at 28 weeks and before delivery.
8. Obstetric problems associated with diabetes include stillbirth, mechanical problems in the birth canal owing to fetal macrosomia (large for gestational dates), hydramnios and pre-eclampsia. Delivery should be in hospital. Pregnancy staging should be assessed using ultrasound. Caesarian section is often required.

Planning a Pregnancy

Diabetes pregnancy carries a risk of congenital malformations and that risk can be restricted by appropriate planning of the pregnancy. Ideally this should take place in a combined clinic attended by a range of relevant health care professionals. Planning encompasses: contraception; drug therapy; metabolic control; smoking and alcohol; vitamin folate supplements. Contraception has been discussed above but in patients with hypertension and cardiovascular disease particular care should be taken with combined oestrogen-progesterone therapy. Angiotensin converting enzyme inhibitors and statins should be stopped and perhaps the former replaced with methyldopa, established to be safe. Smoking should be stopped and alcohol intake limited to restrict fetal risk. Rubella immunity should be assessed and sickle and thalassaemia-trait determined in the woman and, if positive, her partner. Finally, there is evidence that high-dose folate supplementation pre-pregnancy reduces the risk of the congenital malformation due to neural tube defects.

Table 2 **Diabetic control in the first trimester**

HbA1c	Major congenital abnormalities	Total number of deliveries
< 8.5	2	58
> 8.5	13	58

Source: Miller E, Hare JW, Cloherty JP 1981. Elevated maternal haemoglobin A1 in early pregnancy and major congenital malformations in infants of diabetic mothers. N Engl J Med. 304: 1331–4.

Table 3 **Management plan of diabetes in the three trimesters**

Trimester	Management
First	Folate supplements (to reduce congenital malformation risk) Stop smoking, limit alcohol Optimum diabetes control Screen for diabetes complications Ultrasound scan (for fetal congenital anomalies)
Second	Stop smoking, limit alcohol Optimum diabetes control (insulin dose increases) Screen and treat diabetes complications Monitor and treat blood pressure Ultrasound scan (for fetal congenital anomalies, growth)
Third	Stop smoking, limit alcohol Optimum diabetes control (insulin dose increases to 34-36 weeks) Screen and treat diabetes complications Monitor and treat blood pressure Check for pre-eclampsia (twice as common as normal) Ultrasound scan (for fetal congenital anomalies, growth) Plan delivery

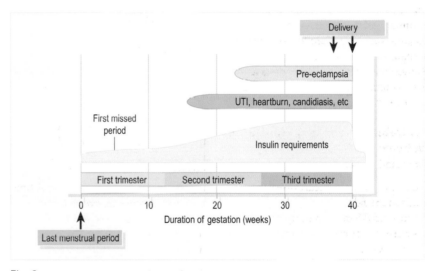

Fig. 2 **Impact of diabetes on the mother.**

Problems in neonates and children

Fetal and neonatal problems

Maternal diabetes, especially when poorly controlled, is associated with fetal macrosomia (Fig. 1) and accelerated fetal growth (Fig. 2). The infant of a diabetic mother is more susceptible to hyaline membrane disease (a disease of the lung membrane that causes respiratory distress) than non-diabetic infants of similar maturity and to congenital malformations. These abnormalities are principally related to hyperglycaemia, congenital malformations being largely determined by hyperglycaemia in the first trimester (see Table 2, p. 103).

Common major congenital malformations seen in infants of diabetic mothers are:

- cardiac
  - great vessel anomalies
  - septal defects

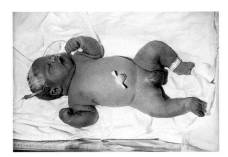

Fig. 1 **Macrosomia in a baby with a diabetic mother.**

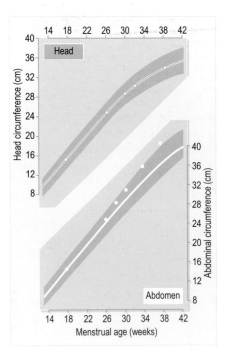

Fig. 2 **Accelerated fetal growth.** The line represents the 50th centile and the shaded area 3rd to 97th centile.

- central nervous system
  - ancephaly
  - spina bifida
- skeletal and facial
  - caudal regression syndrome (Fig. 3)
  - cleft palate or lip
  - arthrogryposis (Fig. 4)
- genitourinary tract
  - renal agenesis
  - ureteric duplication.

Management

The management of a pregnant diabetic mother needs to be carefully planned (see Table 3, p. 103). Ultrasound scanning should be carried out in each trimester; in the first to assess for congenital anomalies and in the second

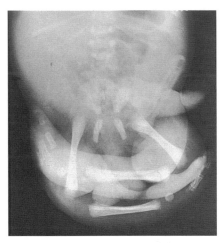

Fig. 3 **Caudal regression and sacral agenesis in a child of a diabetic mother.**

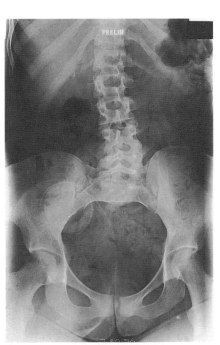

Fig. 4 **Hemivertebra, causing spinal distortion, another mid-line congenital lesion in infants associated with diabetes in the mother.**

and third to assess for congenital anomalies and growth rate.

Labour and delivery

Labour and delivery are potentially hazardous for the diabetic mother and her baby. The delivery should be carefully planned based on the assessment of the fetus during gestation. The need for Caesarean section should be constantly reviewed and is used more frequently in diabetics. Indications for elective delivery by the abdomen include:

- malpresentation
- disproportion between child and birth canal
- intrauterine growth retardation
- fetal distress
- pre-eclampsia.

Diabetes control is by diet or insulin. Insulin requirements are low during labour and insulin can be given by continuous intravenous insulin infusion (typically 2–4 U/h of fast-acting soluble insulin) plus 10% glucose infusion at 125 mL/h (i.e. 1 litre every 8 hours) with regular blood glucose (usually capillary sample) monitoring. After delivery, the insulin requirements fall to prepregnancy levels and the insulin infusion rate should be reduced by half initially.

Immediate neonatal period

Neonatal hypoglycaemia may occur in infants born to a diabetic mother. The neonatal hypoglycaemia occurs because maternal glucose crosses the placenta, but insulin does not; the fetal islets hypersecrete insulin to combat the hyperglycaemia of maternal origin. When the umbilical cord is severed, the neonatal glucose falls to hypoglycaemic levels. Other problems in neonates include:

- respiratory distress syndrome (uncommon now)
- transient hypertrophic cardiomyopathy (30% affected on ultrasound)
- hypocalcaemia (50%)
- hypomagnesaemia (80%)
- polycythaemia (12%)
- jaundice (60%).

Children

Most children with diabetes have type 1 diabetes mellitus but a proportion have maturity-onset diabetes of the young (MODY; see Table 1, p. 62). The former

Table 1 **Principal causes of diabetes mellitus in childhood**

Type	Causes
Type 1	Autoimmune (p. 60)
Maturity-onset diabetes of the young (MODY)	Dominantly inherited variant of type 2 (see p. 63)
Type 2	
Secondary diabetes	
Chromosomal abnormalities:	Down's syndrome
	Turner's syndrome
	Klinefelter's syndrome
Inherited disorders	Prader–Willi syndrome
	Laurence–Moon–Biedl syndrome
	DIDMOAD syndrome
	Leprechaunism
	Lipodystrophy
	Ataxia-telangiectasia
	(Rabson) Mendenhall syndrome
Inherited disorder with pancreatic disease	Cystic fibrosis
Postpancreatectomy	Cystinosis
	Thalassaemia

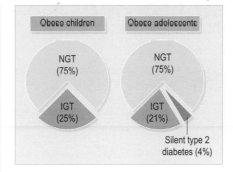

Fig. 5 **Prevalence of type 2 diabetes and glucose intolerance in obese children and adolescents.** NGT, normal glucose tolerance; IGT, impaired glucose tolerance.

are invariably treated with insulin, the latter often manage on diet or tablets. The physician should be alerted to the possibility of MODY when there is a strong family history of diabetes. The increase in childhood obesity in one reason for the increase in type 2 diabetes and glucose intolerance in youth (Fig. 5).

Management

Management of children is not unlike management of the adult. However it often requires particular sensitivity to the childs' social independence and social dependency. These parameters vary with age, the latter being more acute in adolescence, the former more relevant in infancy.

Hypoglycaemia is a particular problem in children in whom the warning symptoms can differ from those in adults. Symptoms of note in children caused by hypoglycaemia include:

- bed-wetting
- naughtiness
- tearfulness
- bad temper
- poor performance in school.

Hyperglycaemia targets should be the same as adult patients (Table 1, p. 88). Sometimes the fear of hypoglycaemia limits attempts to obtain optimum diabetes control. If optimum control is difficult, any reduction in HbA1c is associated with a marked decrease in complication risk. Therefore, attempts should always be continued to achieve better control.

Box 1 lists common questions regarding children with diabetes.

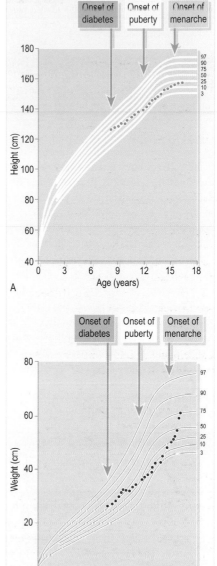

Fig. 6 **Centile growth charts for height (a) and weight (b) for a girl who developed diabetes at 8 years of age.** Puberty and menarche were slightly delayed.

Box 1 Common questions regarding children with diabetes

Immunization. Programmes are unaltered for diabetic children.

Ill health. Illness is no more prevalent in diabetic children, though urinary tract infection is more common.

Bed wetting. No more prevalent in diabetic children but might be caused by nocturnal hyperglycaemia or hypoglycaemia.

Injections. Reluctance to take injections should be sympathetically handled and expert advice sought on needleless pens and injection technique.

Hypoglycaemia. May present differently in children to adults. Blood glucose should be measured if there is doubt. People around the child should be aware that the child has diabetes and what to do in case they develop hypoglycaemic coma.

Diet. This should be similar as for the rest of the family, and low in sugar. A routine for meal times should be established as far as possible.

Behaviour and lifestyle. Diabetic children should be expected to participate in all aspects of sport and play at school. Teachers may need to be advised that diabetes is an excellent opportunity for manipulative behaviour. We all do it, but having diabetes is no excuse to live a different life. Naughtiness, tears, bad temper and poor performance in school can be associated with hypoglycaemia.

Growth. On average, growth is minimally reduced in diabetes; reduction can occur particularly in very young children with poor control. Puberty may also be delayed by 2 years or arrested (Fig. 6). Both should be monitored and if changes are noted then referral to a specialist may be required to exclude other causes (e.g. hypothyroidism) and for therapy as required.

Problems in neonates and children

Fetus and neonate

- The infants of diabetic mothers can have macrosomia and accelerated fetal growth, and are more susceptible to congenital abnormalities and hyaline membrane disease.

- Fetal problems are principally related to hyperglycaemia.

- Diabetes management is vital at all periods of pregnancy and includes the prepregnancy planning period and the postnatal phase.

Children

- Most children with diabetes have type 1 diabetes mellitus but MODY and type 2 diabetes also occur.

- Obesity increases risk of glucose intolerance and diabetes.

- Hypoglycaemia may present differently in children to adults.

The elderly and ethnic groups

Elderly people with diabetes mellitus

There is a huge increase in older patients with diabetes mellitus; by 2025, about a third of patients with diabetes mellitus will be aged over age 75 years. This population is at especially high risk of diabetes-related death, macrovascular disease, hypertension and cataracts. In part, the increase in diabetes frequency is caused by age-related changes in glucose metabolism, including decreased insulin secretion and decreased insulin sensitivity (Fig. 1). Prevention and treatment of complications should be as active as in the younger population. Hyperglycaemia is usually caused by type 2 diabetes mellitus, but type 1 diabetes may present at this age.

Approximately 10% of people over 65 years of age have diabetes mellitus that has been diagnosed and another 10% have undiagnosed hyperglycaemia. Clinical presentation in older people is often not as clear-cut as in children and adults. Weight loss in the elderly may be caused by ketoacidosis and need not only be caused by cancer or reduced appetite. Incontinence, immobility or intellectual deterioration could also be caused by diabetes mellitus.

Management

A number of factors in the elderly interfere with compliance and complicate the management of patients. Multiple pathologies and drug therapies can result in drug interactions and poor compliance. Of particular note, the number of drugs is related inversely to compliance. Drugs in the elderly are not metabolized as efficiently as in the young. As a result drug dosages may need to be low or reduced. It may be necessary to identify the most important areas for intervention rather than identify all therapies required.

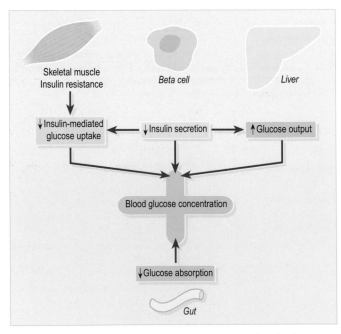

Fig. 1 **Age-related changes in carbohydrate metabolism lead to a raised blood glucose despite reduced glucose absorption.**

Management problems with diabetes mellitus in the elderly include:

- living alone, poverty, poor diet: poor compliance
- intellectual impairment, depression and dementia: poor compliance
- poor vision and dexterity: difficulty with blood test and injections
- coexisting diseases and drugs: potential for confusion and drug interaction
- multiple drug therapy: poor compliance
- decreased mobility and exercise: poor lifestyle.

A good approach to therapy of diabetes mellitus in the elderly would include:

- determining current quality of life and prognosis
- assessing priorities in treating diabetes and other diseases
- avoiding hypoglycaemia
- treating diabetes mellitus according to individual targets
- screening for complications and treating to maintain quality of life
- being cautious with drug dosages and insulin use.

Management of risk factors in the elderly

Management of the elderly is not unlike management of the child requiring the same sensitivity to individual social independence and social dependency.

Hypoglycaemia is a particular problem in older patients taking oral hypoglycaemic agents. Long acting sulphonylureas, such as chlorpropamide and glibenclamide, are particularly likely to cause severe attacks because of poor clearance; these should be avoided in patients over age 65 years of age.

Hyperglycaemia targets should be the same as for other patients (Table 1, p. 88). Even if optimum control is difficult, any reduction in HbA1c is associated with a marked decrease in complication risk.

The short-acting meglitinides such as repaglinide and nateglinide are less likely to cause hypoglycaemia than chlorpropamide or glibenclamide. Non-insulinotropic agents, such as metformin, acarbose or thiazolidinediones, are potentially safer in that they do not cause hypoglycaemia. However each of these agents is associated with other side-effects. Metformin should be used with caution in patients with impaired renal or cardiac function, because of the rare occurrence of lactic acidosis.

Isolated systolic hypertension is prevalent in the elderly population and more than 70% of adults aged over 64 years can be considered to be hypertensive (systolic BP > or = 140 mmHg and/or diastolic or = 90 mmHg). Systolic pressure is a better predictor of cardiovascular events than diastolic pressure and a wide pulse pressure is a better predictor than either alone. Trials of elderly patients showed clear cardiovascular benefit in treating isolated systolic hypertension. Current recommendations suggest a lowering of systolic blood pressure by no more than 20 mmHg in the first instance to prevent postural hypotension. Particular care should be taken when starting

ACE inhibitors in the elderly as the risk of intolerance due to renovascular disease is appreciable.

All elderly patients are at high risk of macrovascular disease and therefore strong candidates for treatment with both aspirin (at low dose) and with a statin. Contraindications for aspirin include a previous haemorrhage or a peptic ulcer. The evidence in non-diabetic subjects supports the introduction of statins up to the age of 70 years in those at cardiovascular risk which probably includes all diabetes patients age 65 or more. There is a strong case for introducing statins in all elderly diabetes patients where appropriate irrespective of age.

Ethnic groups

Epidemiology

Whilst type 1 diabetes is most prevalent in North America and Europe, type 2 diabetes is most prevalent elsewhere, especially in populations that have only recently been exposed to 'Western' lifestyles. Notable amongst these are North American Indians, Pacific islanders and Australian Aborigines, but also populations such as Indians who have migrated to Europe or North America. The explosion in the global frequency of diabetes predominantly relates to type 2 diabetes and is already evident in parts of Asia, the Middle-East and Central and South America (see p. 62). These changes in diabetes prevalence worldwide have been attributed to the excess consumption of calories allied to the decreased use of them due to reduced physical activity. Of particular note, the disease profile in some populations extends to an association with insulin resistance and macrovascular disease so that Indians and Arabs are prone to heart disease while Native American Indians are not.

As a result, some ethnic groups may require particularly aggressive and early intervention with primary prevention strategies, for example, to reduce blood pressure and improve the lipid profile, though unequivocal evidence for the success of such strategies is awaited.

Patients with diabetes mellitus should be treated in the same manner, irrespective of their race, and according to the type of diabetes and risk factors. However, there are certain features of some ethnic groups that warrant awareness:

- there is wide variation in diabetes mellitus incidence according to race, both for type 1 and type 2
- macrovascular disease is particularly prevalent in some ethnic groups such as Asian Indians. In them, metabolically neutral drugs such as angiotensin-converting enzyme inhibitors and calcium channel blocking agents can be used as first-line agents.
- hyperosmolar non-ketotic coma is more common in African-Americans than in people of European origin
- hypertension in patients of African origin is often associated with low renin, so response to angiotensin-converting enzyme inhibitors is poor: β-adrenoceptor blockers and calcium channel blockers are the first choice (though evidence for the success of this strategy is lacking).

Ramadan

Ramadan (the Muslim holy period when the faithful fast during daylight hours) poses a problem for those on tablets or insulin. During Ramadan, the diet pattern changes. Food is eaten twice per day: at Suhur (before sunrise) and at Iftar (after sunset), but not inbetween those times. Patients with diabetes should take Suhur just before sunrise, and not earlier, and be very strict about avoiding sweet food, instead filling up with rice, chapatti or naan.

It is possible to obtain permission to eat during Ramadan for medical reasons, and patients should consult their holy leader if unsure. Alternatively, during daylight hours, they could avoid short-acting insulinotrophic agents (e.g. sulphonylureas) and insulin itself (e.g. soluble insulin). Hypoglycaemia and dehydration are the main problems. They must break the fast if they feel a hypoglycaemic attack.

Table 1 **Ethnic variation in prevalence of type 2 diabetes in populations aged 30–64 years (World Health Organisation)**

	Prevalence (%)	Risk ratio
Pima Indians	50	12
Peninsular Arabs	25	6
South Asians	20	5
West Africans	12	3
North Americans	7	2
North Europeans	4	1

The elderly and ethnic groups

- Diabetes and impaired glucose tolerance is common in the elderly.
- Management of diabetes in the elderly requires a particularly flexible approach.
- Ethnic differences exist in terms of complication risk and response to certain therapy.
- Ramadan for the Muslim faith requires counselling to avoid hypoglycaemia during daylight.

Index